The Five Minute Face Lift Workout

How Five Minutes of Simple Exercises Once a Day Can Make You Look Years Younger

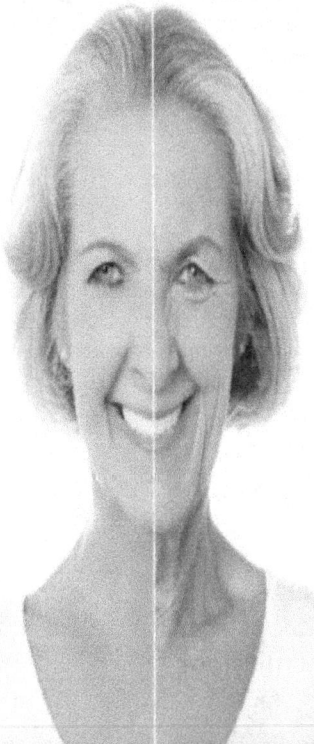

Smooth Frown Lines

Fade Crow's Feet

Deflate Eye Bags

Lift Droopy Eye Lids

Accentuate Cheeks

Erase Turkey Neck

Prevent 'Misery Mouth'

Anti-Aging Secrets

The Easy Non-Surgical Face Lift

The Five Minute Face Lift Workout:

How Five Minutes of Simple, Easy-to-Learn Exercises Could Make You Look Ten Years Younger

ISBN: 978-1-291-71636-8

Goodall Copywriting
Pyewell Cottage
The Green
Westerham
Kent
TN16 1AS
Great Britain

www.goodallcopywriting.com

http://www.goodallcopywriting.com/face-lift-workout 2

Acknowledgements

I would like to thank Jan, Jane, Jim, David, Kit and Phil for their help and encouragement in making the seed of an idea become ink, paper and pdf.

Several experts in the field of health, nutrition and fitness have kindly allowed me to include their material in this book.

My appreciation is also extended to Hypnosis Downloads for their insights into the power of the subconscious mind, eVitamins whose wide and detailed knowledge of natural healthcare and disease prevention has made an invaluable contribution, Penis Advantage for their detailed knowledge of how to improve on what God gave us and Animal Aid for the use of their dietary information.

Lastly, my thanks to Myrna for proof-reading this work and saving me from lexicon-induced embarrassment.

For more information about these contributors go to:

animalaid.org

The Face Lift Workout Works!

Here is what others are saying about The Five Minute Face Lift Workout non-surgical face lift exercise system you will find inside:

" I think this is really good. I love your exercises." SB.

"Simon- these are really terrific exercises & you explain them & demonstrate them easy & in a timely manner...unlike some others on you tube that go on & on. you are succinct & to the point!!! so appreciated. Thanx again! I tried this & the jowl one. they are both excellent. I can really feel a burn when doing them so I know they are working/engaging the muscles. I will try the others too! keep up the good work. Thanx." Bijouxzane.

"Thanks Simon!! Looking forward to getting your book and learning more techniques." John L.

"Thank you for that short and excellent workout, my neck looks good already." 958ball.

"Hello Simon, i must say u have a cute face, i am getting results already, thank you so much for taking your time to show these quick and simple exercises. " An Admirer.

"Thank you so much,i been looking for this answer for a long time and now i know how to exercise? eye muscles your are my hero ." Khaamkhuu Cabdulaahi

http://www.goodallcopywriting.com/face-lift-workout 4

"Just tried this and my cheek muscles feel like they have been to the gym.. thanks Simon. :)" Pagani Zonda

"Very clear, concise and easy to do. You really feel it afterwards, thanks for explaining how to do it so well too." cleanfreak73.

"It works!!!" 65watchman.

"Thank you, so much I already see good changes." Angel S.

"I love your new product The Five Minute Face Lift Workout and I think your perspective on the matter is really unique. I really think The Five Minute Face Lift Workout for Men is one of the best products in its market. Congratulations and keep up the great work." Ovi Dogar.

Introduction

Hello, my name is Simon and I am a freelance writer.

Writing articles for magazines and on-line
has led me down some interesting lines
of research and none have been so fascinating
as the subject of health and fitness and how it
can keep us looking and feeling younger
for longer.

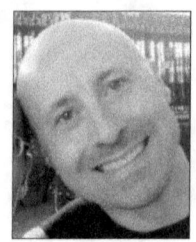

This book explores the many well-researched and thoroughly tested ways you can slow down and even reverse the signs of aging, whether it be through exercise, a change of diet, sex-boosting natural aphrodisiacs, beauty secrets or unleashing the infinite power of your subconscious mind.

No-one is ever going to completely beat Father Time, but if you integrate these anti-aging techniques into your life, you can certainly give him a good run for his money.

Simon
January 2016

The Five Minute Face Lift Workout

Go into any newsagent or magazine seller and you will see a wide selection of well-known fitness publications. The glossy covers show young people with beautiful bodies and their pages will be packed full of conventional exercise regimes designed to strengthen and tone nearly every muscle in your body.

Without doubt these workout routines will keep your body strong, healthy and more resilient to disease, in fact, I've included my own 'fast fitness' exercise routine in this book because regular exercise is a vital weapon in your quest to stay sexy.

While these magazines concentrate on the body, very much less is said about another, neglected set of muscles that have a huge impact on how young or old you look and feel - the muscles in our face.

Yet, while the muscles in the body are exercised almost to obsession, those in the face are usually neglected and left to wither away. It is this deterioration in the tone and strength of the facial muscles that encourages the formation of wrinkles, sunken eyes, hollow cheeks, eye bags and a flabby neck.

Without toned muscles to support the skin, gravity sucks your features down, making you look drawn and tired. The corners of the mouth droop downwards giving you with a permanently sad expression.

You may think that because you use the muscles in your face every day to talk, eat and make expressions, this would be enough to keep them in good condition but this type of sporadic, uncoordinated movement is not enough to keep the facial muscles in their best condition.

We assume that this deterioration in our looks is just a natural part of the aging process but I disagree. Many women have known for a long time that simple daily exercises that tone the major facial muscle groups can help to firm the contours of the face and prevent or reduce the visible signs of aging.

Just as with the muscles of the body, if you exercise the muscles in your face, you can stay looking fresher and younger for longer.
The idea of exercising the muscles of your face may seem a little strange but it can become a normal and natural part of your daily routine and it only need take 5 minutes a day.

No matter what your age you can look and feel better with facial exercise. If you are young, performing facial exercises will help you maintain that smooth, fresh, healthy look of youth. If you are more mature, a facial workout will help 'turn back the clock'.

Performed regularly, facial exercises can:

■   Firm the forehead, reducing worry and frown lines;

■   Reduce and prevent crows feet and bags around the eyes;

■   Stop the downward turn of your mouth and thinning of the

lips;

■   Accentuate your cheekbones to give a more elegant tapered shape to the face;

■   Reduce and prevent jowls and slack neck skin (turkey neck);

■   Fill out the sides of the mouth to prevent hollow cheeks.

This step-by-step guide shows you easy-to-learn, simple exercises that will give you a natural, non-surgical face lift and it's guaranteed to work for you, regardless of your age.

The Muscles of the Face

There are sixteen major groups of muscles that influence how the face looks. The diagram below shows a simplified view of how the facial muscles are arranged on the skull and the legend on the next page gives the name of each muscle group.

As you will see, muscles cover almost the entire face and head and therefore have a huge influence on your unique appearance.

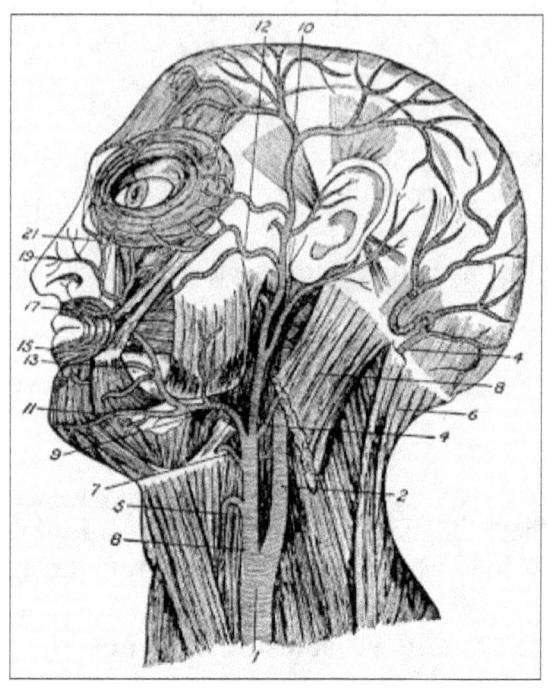

1, longus colli; 2, rapezius; 3, sterno-hyoid; 4, sterno-mastoid; 5, erico-thyroid; 6, trapezius; 7, constrictor of pharynx; 8, sterno-mastoid; 9, digastric; 10, attrahens aurem; 11, mylo-hyoid; 12, masseter; 13, depressor of lower lip; 15, orbicularis oris; 17, levator of upper lip; 19, levator of angle of mouth; 21, orbicularis palpebrarum. Source: Joseph G. Richardson, Health and Longevity (New York, Home Health Society, 1912).

The following exercises, if performed correctly and regularly, will tone and strengthen these major facial muscles, restoring their tone and strength.

Each exercise is clearly explained in words and pictures and you also have the option of watching a demonstration video.

You will be exercising your muscles 'isometrically'. This means you will be tensing the muscles against counter pressure from your hands for a number of seconds and then relaxing.

At first it may seem very difficult to perform each exercise or to feel any effect. This is normal. Much like the muscles of your body, any exercise performed for the first time on muscles that have not been actively exercised for years will be a challenge.

Even holding the tension for a few seconds may seem impossible but don't give up! When you first work out the biceps on your arms it can be difficult to even lift the dumbbell off the ground, but the more you do it the stronger the arms muscles become and the easier it gets to lift the dumbbell. It's no different with the muscles in the face.

In the beginning, aim to hold the tension in each muscle for a slow count of 10. Do this every day for one or two months. As the muscles begin to tone and the exercise feels easier, double the tension hold to 20 seconds for another couple of months.

When this becomes comfortable increase the hold to thirty seconds for each exercise.

The important thing is not to rush and expect instant results. Muscle toning takes time, dedication and patience but the rewards are worth the wait and the effort. You don't have to perform all the exercises in one session. If there is a particular part of your face you wish to concentrate on that's fine or you can spread the exercises out over an entire day or week, but for the fastest results and a complete 'makeover' I suggest doing the entire workout on a daily basis.

Before you start make sure your hands are clean and dry so that you can hold the skin under your hands and fingers. If your hands or face are too greasy you may find it hard to create the resistance needed for your facial muscles to work against. If you wash your face before the session, either use a non-drying facial cleanser that does not leave your skin feeling tight or moisturize after your wash with a light, easily absorbed non-greasy lotion or cream and give it time to absorb.

You want your skin to be dry enough so that your fingers and hands do not slip over the skin. You want to be able to hold the skin gently but firmly and work the muscles underneath against that hold.

The Exercises

Each exercise is clearly explained. Please follow the step by step instructions to make sure you perform each exercise correctly. It may be a good idea to practice each exercise in front of a mirror or web cam to check the position of your hands. As you become more confident in performing each exercise you should be able to perform the exercises by feel alone but you can, of course, continue to use a mirror if you wish.

Firming and Smoothing the Forehead

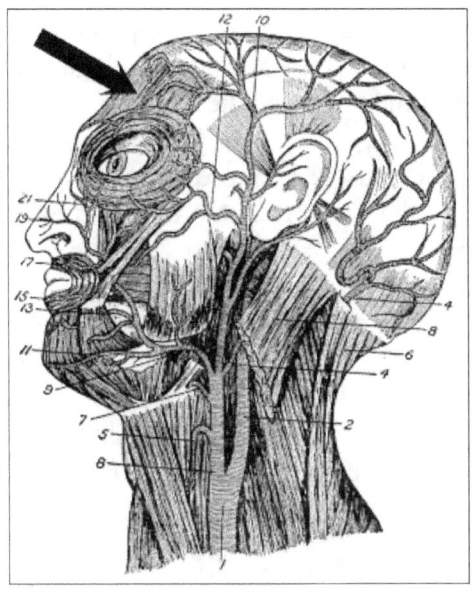

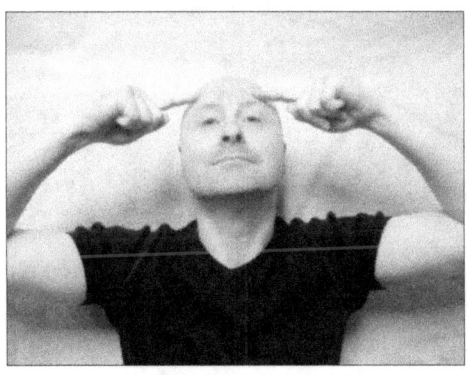

The forehead is covered by a thin sheet of muscle called the occipital frontalis. When you raise your eyebrows, this is the muscle you use. It is also connected to the muscles around the eyes. As we age, this muscle loses it's tone and elasticity, encouraging both frown lines and drooping of the skin over the eyes.

By exercising this muscle, you help smooth and minimize frown lines, lift the eye brows into an elegant arch and prevent the drooping of the upper eye lid.

As the forehead muscle increases in tone, you should feel the tension across the front of your forehead when you perform this exercise.

Place both palms of the hands over the forehead, so that the fingers rest on the front of your head and scalp, and your thumbs touch your temples. The lower part of your palms covers your eyebrows. Press your palms firmly against the forehead bone and gently pull the skin upwards and outwards.

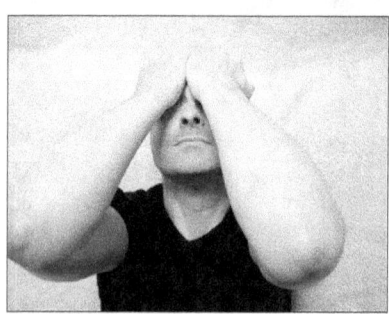 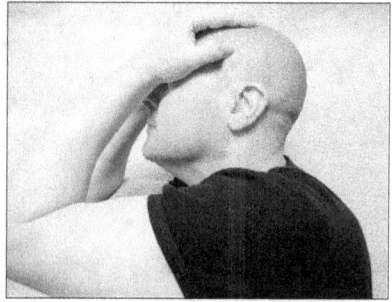

Use your palms to provide resistance. Place your palms over your forehead. Now slowly pull your eye brows and forehead down, trying to close your eyes against the upper pressure of your palms. Try to move the entire sheath of muscle across your forehead down towards your nose. Try not to frown or use only the eyebrows. Use your palms to keep your eyebrows gently separated by pressing outward as well as upward.

You should feel tension across your forehead only. Hold the tension for a slow count of up to 30 seconds, then gently drop the forehead skin down to it's resting position, release the tension and take away your palms. Do this once a day.

Eyes

The eyes are surrounded by a muscle called the orbicularis occuli. When you squint in strong sunlight or close your eyes tightly, you are using this muscle. As the muscles becomes weak and flaccid, the eyes can start to look droopy, crows feet can form at the edge of each eye and eye bags can appear.

The following three exercises help to tone the upper, side and lower parts of the eye muscle in isolation, for a more alert, awake and bright eyed expression.

> For more anti-aging tips go to goodallcopywriting.com and visit the blog.

Upper Eyes/Eye Lids

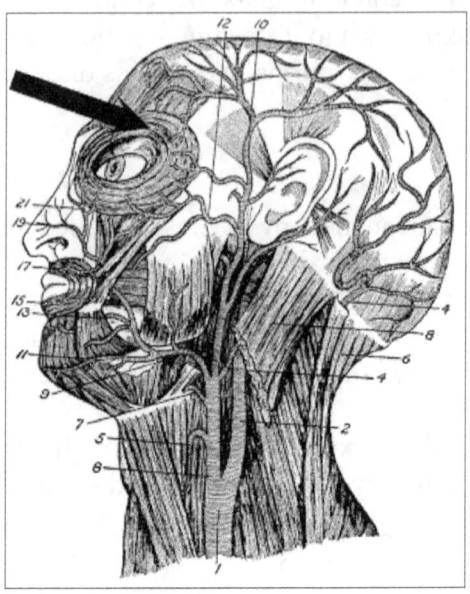

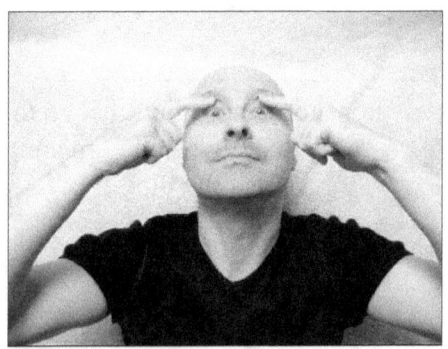

As this muscle gains tone, you should feel tension across the upper part of your eyes, between the eyebrows and eyelids.

Place the thumbs of each hand against the upper eye sockets, under your eye brows, with your fingers placed on either side of your head.

Press gently upwards against the upper eye socket bone to provide resistance and now try to close the lids of your eyelids. Your eyelids may flutter with the exertion as you slowly try to close them. It may help to look downwards with your eyes while you perform this exercise. Feel the tension between your eyebrows and upper eye lids only.

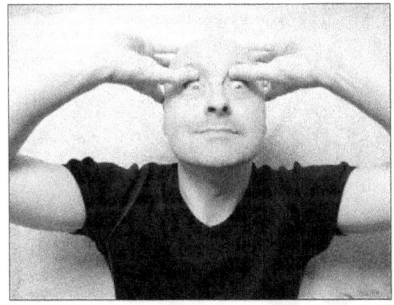 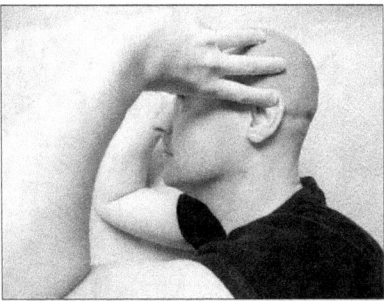

Hold for a count of up 30 seconds then slowly release the tension. Do this once a day.

For more anti-aging tips go to goodallcopywriting.com and visit the blog.

Side of Eyes

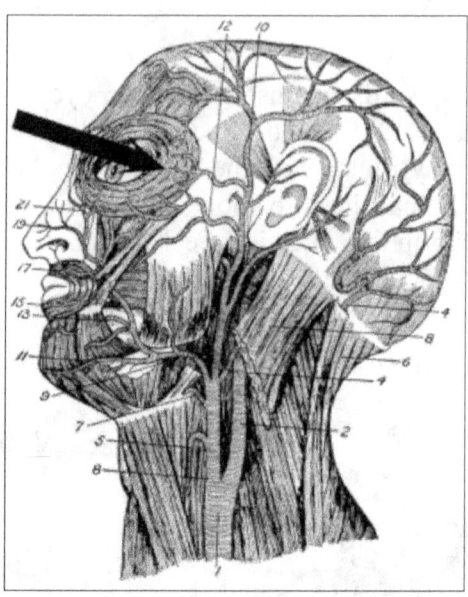

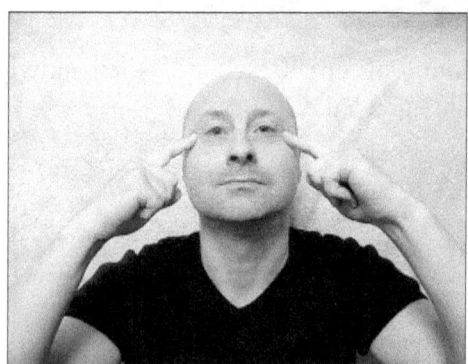

This exercise will tone the small muscle at the side of your eyes to reduce crows feet and prevent new ones forming.

Place the index finger of each hand at the outer edge of the lower eye socket.

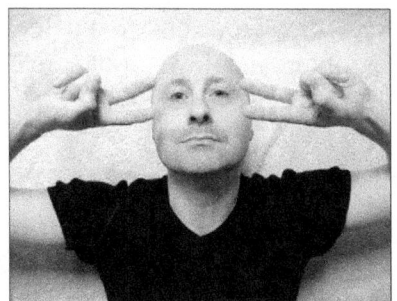 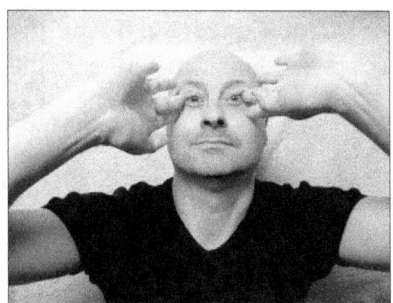

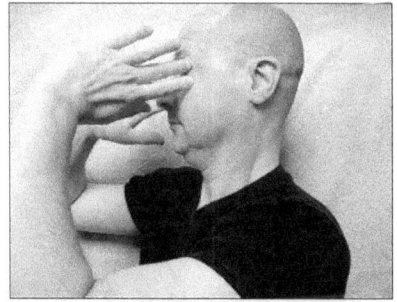

Place the middle finger at the outer edge of the upper eye socket, just below the outer eyebrow. Both fingers should form a horizontal V at right angles to your face. Press the fingers of each hand gently against the bone of the outer eye socket and provide resistance by gently separating your fingers.

Now slowly try to squint, using the outer eye muscle only, against the resistance of your fingers gently pushing apart. Do not shut your eyes, keep them open and looking straight ahead. If you can shut them, you are not providing enough resistance with your fingers.

Hold for up to a slow count of 30, then slowly relax the tension.

Do this once a day. As the muscles develop, you should feel strong tension between the upper outer and lower outer eye socket.

Lower Eyes

This exercise will tone the sheath of eye muscle that runs under your eye, between the lower eye lid and the lower eye socket. Toning this muscle can help reduce and prevent eye bags.

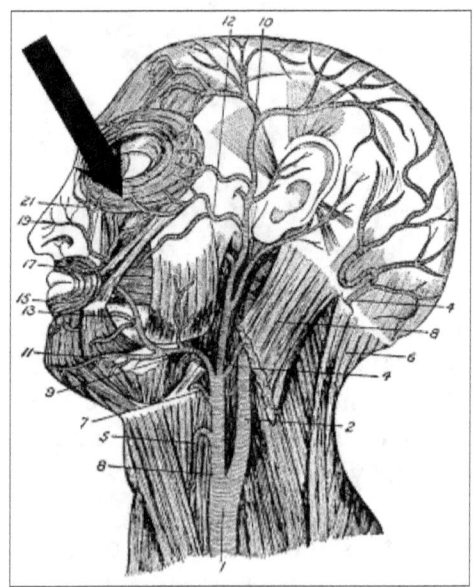

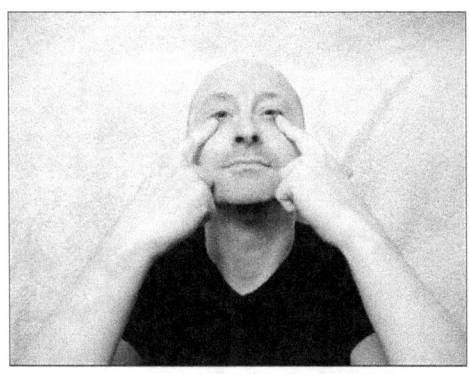

Place the index finger of each hand against the bone of the upper eye socket below your eyebrows and the middle finger just below the bone of the lower eye socket, above each cheek. Place you thumbs on the side of your face, near the front of your ears, for support. Your fingers should form a wide, horizontal V shape in front of your eyes.

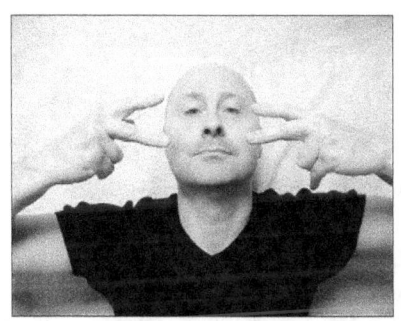 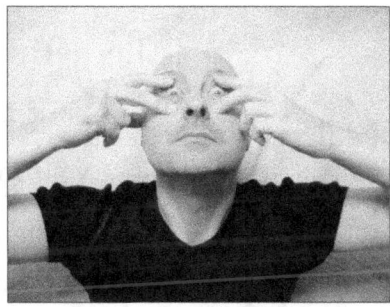

Press gently against the eye socket bone to provide resistance. Now try to close your eyes, or squint against the resistance of your fingers. Keep your eyes open and looking straight ahead. You will also feel tension at the side of your eyes as the ring of muscle surrounding each eye tenses up.

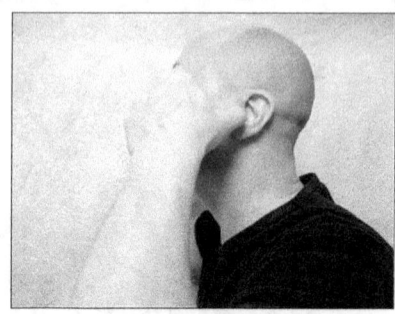

Keep the rest of the face relaxed apart from the lower eye muscle. Try not to frown or furrow your brow while you hold the tension. Hold for a slow count of up to 30, then slowly relax the tension.

As the muscle tones up, you should feel tension around the entire eye but especially in the area between your lower finger and the lower eye lid.

Alternative Technique

A different way to achieve the same effect on your eyes is to use the outside edge of your forefingers and thumbnail side of your thumbs as anchors.

Place your forefingers just under your upper eye socket and the thumbnail side of your thumbs on top of your lower eye socket.

Press your fingers gently onto the upper and lower eye sockets and then try to close your eyes.

Don't just use your eye lids to close your eyes, squint your eyes closed. You should feel a tightening effect on both the upper and lower eye muscles.

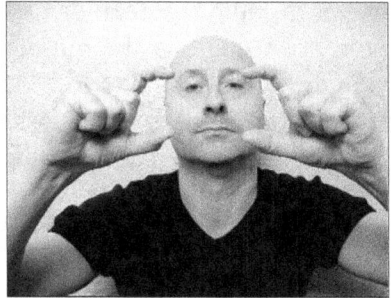 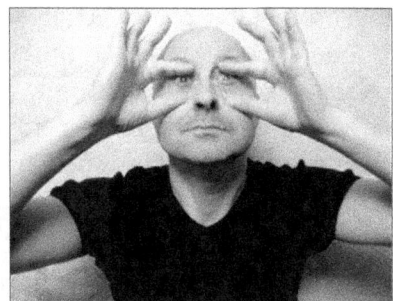

For more anti-aging tips go to
goodallcopywriting.com and
visit the blog.

Lips

There is a circular band of muscle that surrounds the lips called the orbicularis oris. Clench your lips tightly together or say "Ooooo" and this is the muscle you are using. As the muscle wastes away the lips become thin and the mouth starts to turn downwards, giving a permanent expression of sadness. Keeping this muscle toned will keep the shape of the mouth and prevent wrinkles forming at the side of the mouth.

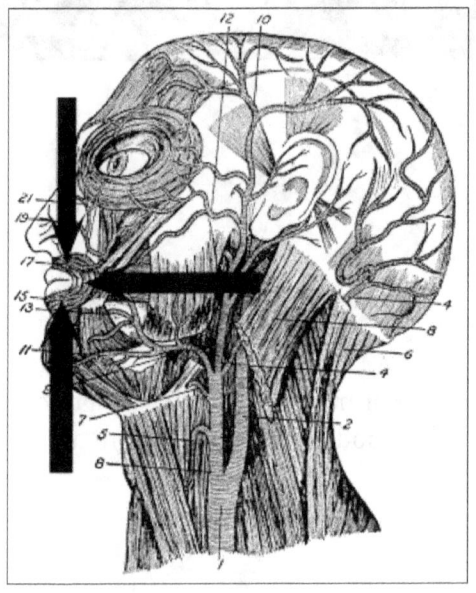

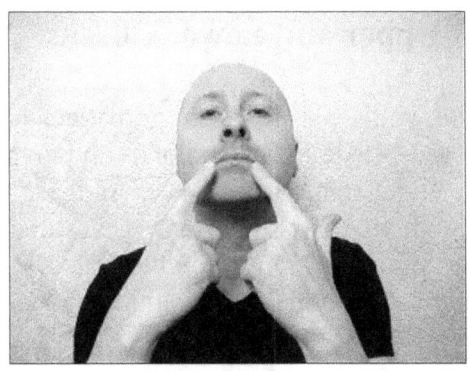

Put the fingers of your left or right palm together and tilt your hand horizontally. Place your forefinger side of the palm between your lips.

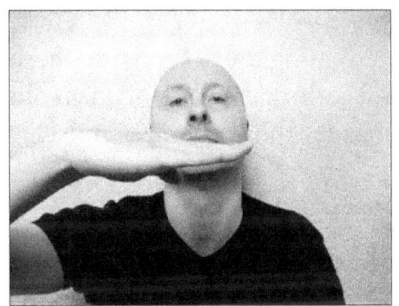 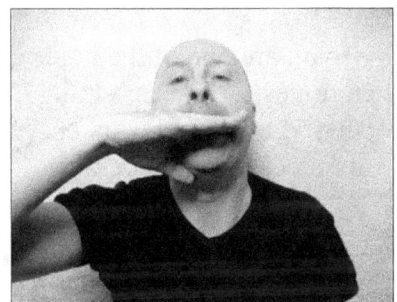

Press your lips down onto your finger. Keep your lips tucked back against your teeth during the exercise and try not to wrinkle your nose or pout.

Work just the mouth muscles in isolation. Hold the tension up to the count of 30 then slowly relax. As the muscle develops you should feel a ring of tension around your lips as you perform the exercise.

Upper and Lower Cheeks

When you smile, you are using the zygomaticus major muscles and these help accentuate the cheekbones and give a tapered or upside down triangle shape to the face. As these muscles also help lift the mouth when smiling, toning up these muscles not only adds shape and definition to the face but also counter-acts the natural downward droop of the mouth.

Exercising these muscles can be easy or more challenging depending on how you use your face when talking. Some people's faces are very animated when they talk and use these muscles a lot. Others tend to only move the mouth when talking while the rest of the face stays still.

If you are one of the latter group, isolating and exercising these muscles will seem strange, but the effort is worth it to avoid that drawn and sunken look a face full of slack muscles assumes as time goes by.

Upper Cheeks

Try to smile without curling up the sides of your mouth. Feel the muscles pulling your mouth up and out? These are the muscles you will be exercising.

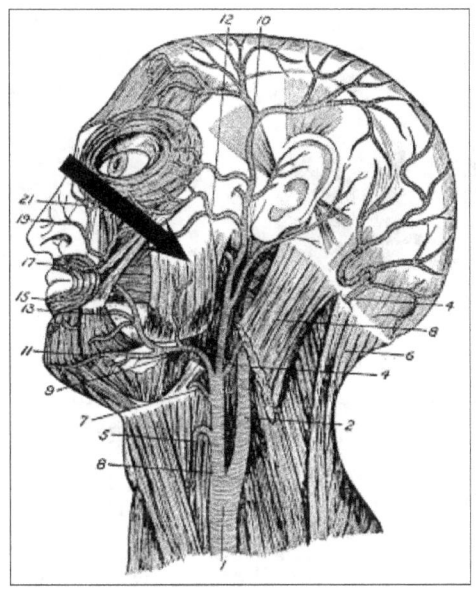

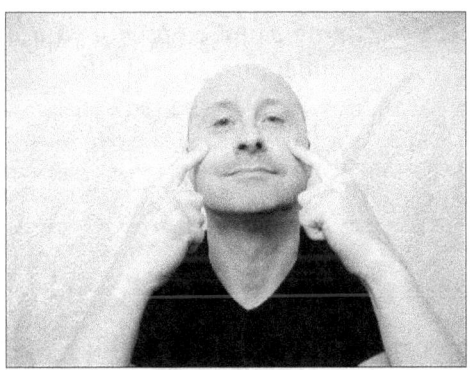

Place the thumbs of each hand under each cheek bone and the other fingers on the side of the head to anchor the thumbs.

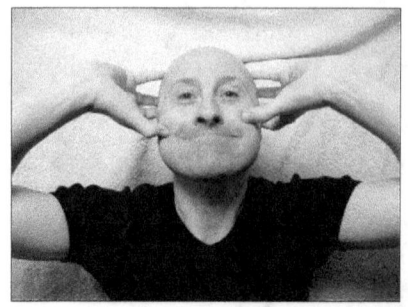 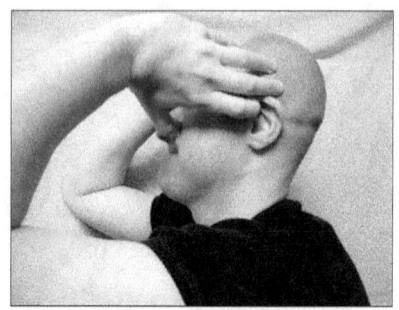

You need to avoid 'snarling' when you perform this exercise as this will encourage lines to run from the edge of your nose to the corners of your mouth. To stop this, gently bite your upper lip and suck it against your teeth. You should also try to avoid squinting with your eyes. Try to isolate the upper cheek muscles only and keep your eyes wide open. Now try to lift your upper cheeks upward and outwards towards your ears.

You should feel your thumbs move up with your cheek muscles as the muscle moves under the skin. Hold for up to a slow count of 30 and then slowly relax the tension.

For more anti-aging tips go to
goodallcopywriting.com and
visit the blog.

Lower Cheeks

This exercise tones up the muscle that form the 'walls' of your mouth and cheeks between your cheekbone and lower jaw. It can help give the face a fuller appearance.

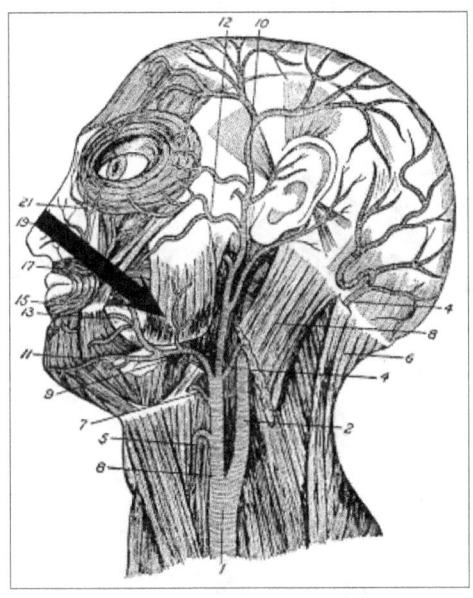

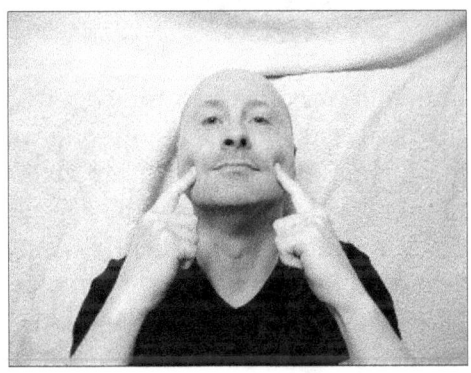

Place the first and middle finger of your right hand together, as if you were making your hand into an upside-down 'gun'.

Your finger nails are facing you and your palms are facing away from you.

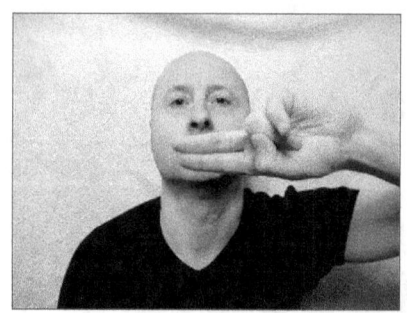 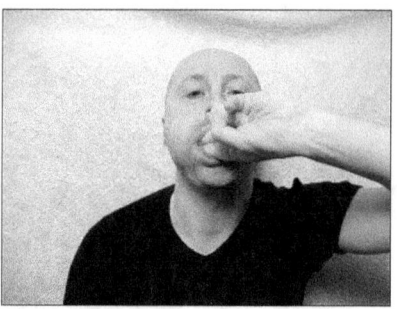

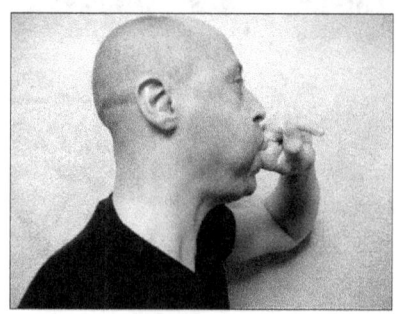

Open your mouth and place the two fingers of your right hand in your mouth, between your teeth/jaw and your left inner cheek. Hold the fingers in your mouth my clamping down on them with your lips. This also tones the muscles around the mouth. Now push your fingers gently away from your teeth/jaw but at the same time try to push your fingers back against your jaw with the muscles in the cheek. Try not to squint the eyes when performing this exercise.

Keep the tension isolated to your lower cheeks only. Hold for a slow count of up to 30 and then slowly relax. Repeat this exercise with your left hand on the opposite right cheek.

The Neck

There is a group of muscles that run from under the chin and jaw bones down to the front and side of the throat. These keep the skin tucked tightly under the jaw. As these muscles lose their tone, folds of skin known as 'turkey neck' can form and so can a double chin. Keeping these muscles strong and toned will help preserve the definition of the chin and jaw.

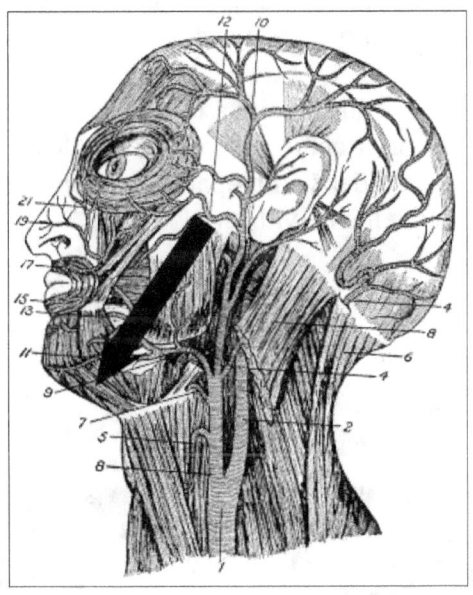

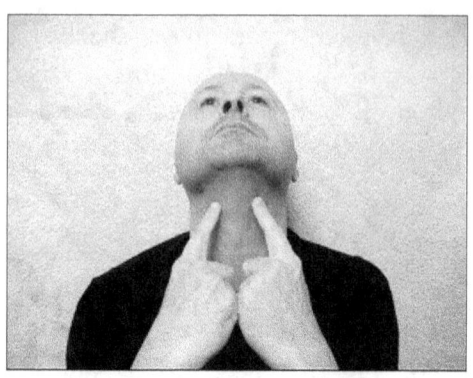

As the muscle develops you should feel the muscles tense from under your chin down the front of your throat, under each jaw running down your neck, and in the large muscles at each side of your throat that support the head.

Find a sturdy table or desk with a top that is roughly just below chest height. Sit on a chair in front of the desk and rest your elbows about a shoulder width apart. Place one fist in the other (it doesn't matter which) with the knuckles of the upper hand facing upwards.

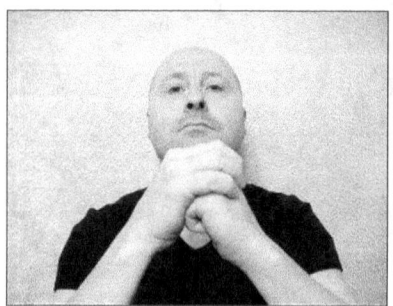 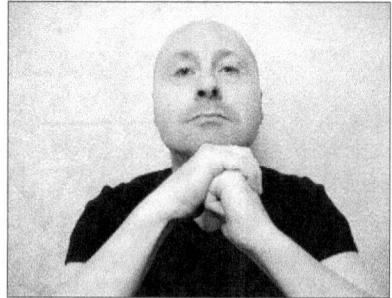

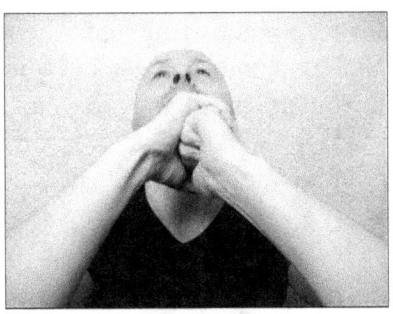

Now rest your chin in the cleft between the first and second knuckle of the upper hand, facing forward. Lean your head back slightly and make sure your teeth are clenched together. Now push your head back down and forward against your anchored fists and arms.

Keep looking forward by pushing your chin forward at the same time you push down against your fists.

Try not to let your chin pivot on your knuckles so you begin to look down. You need to keep the muscle under your chin stretched out and under tension.

Hold for up to 30 seconds and then slowly relax. If you do not have a suitable desk you can push down with your neck against the counter upward pressure of your clenched fists and arms.

As you can see, with these exercises we have worked our way from the top of the face right down to the bottom, giving all the major facial muscles a workout.

Over the coming months you should notice your whole face begin to 'lift', look fuller and more alert. Try taking a photograph of your face before you begin the regime and a few months later. I believe and hope you will see a pleasing difference. When you do, send in your pictures and tell me your story of success. I will place it on the website to encourage others to give the workout a try.

For more anti-aging tips go to goodallcopywriting.com and visit the blog.

The Secrets to Younger Looking Skin

There's no doubt that having smooth, healthy-looking skin goes a long way to making us look and feel younger. Unfortunately, many of us suffer from common skin problems such as lines and wrinkles, dry skin, spots or acne, shaving rash and greasy skin.

There are hundreds of skin problem-solving creams and lotions to choose from, all claiming to be the one you need to give you the beautiful skin you've always wanted but how can you be sure that those magic ingredients will do what they promise?

As well as performing The Five Minute Face Lift Workout every day, it is important to keep your facial skin moisturized with a good quality, vegetable based cream or lotion.

Adding certain essential oils and other plant extracts that have a reputation for their beneficial effects will help to keep your skin looking smooth, clear and fresh.

The next few pages will detail the essential oils I feel you need to include in your skin care routine simply because their benefits have been observed over a long period of time.

Flick through any lifestyle magazine and you will see dozens of full page, glossy advertisements for the latest 'wonder cream'. The marketing text will boast that the cream contains some new, miracle ingredient whose rejuvenating properties can be yours.

One way is to opt for a product that contains ingredients that have been used for hundreds, even thousands of years to help keep skin young looking and healthy.

Even today, practitioners around the globe use the natural plant extracts you will read about in this chapter to minimize the formation of wrinkles and keep skin looking fresh and healthy. There are a number of plant oils that have been proven to deeply penetrate the skin and rejuvenate it from within.

These oils are not like the vegetable or mineral oils you find in shop-bought cosmetics. Their texture is so fine and light they look and feel more like water than oil and it is these bio-active liquids that are the essential ingredient in a branch of herbal medicine called aromatherapy.

Aromatherapy is the therapeutic use of plant-based bio-active substances from flowers, trees, shrubs, leaves, stems, roots and fruits for psychological and physical well-being and it can take many pounds of plant material to make up just one tiny bottle 10 ml of concentrated oil.

Although the word 'aromatherapy' was only coined fairly recently, it has its origins in the most ancient of healing practices, for the plants from which we obtain essential oils have been used in one form or another since man first became aware that he could use plants to heal.

A French chemist by the name of René-Maurice Gattefossé became interested in the use of essential oils for their medicinal use in the early 20th century. Previously, he focused on the aromatic use of essential oils, but his interest in their medicinal use grew after an accident heightened his curiosity. While working, he burned his arm rather badly. By reflex, he plunged his burned arm into the closest liquid which happened to be a large container of lavender essential oil. The burn he suffered healed quickly and left no scar.

Gattefossé is credited with coining the now familiar term of 'aromatherapy' in 1928 in an article he wrote supporting the use of using essential oils in their whole without breaking them down into their primary constituents. .

Robert B. Tisserand is a English aromatherapist who is responsible for being the first individual to bring knowledge and education of aromatherapy to English speaking nations. He has written books and articles including the highly respected 1977 publication The Art of Aromatherapy - the first aromatherapy book published in English.

From the late 20th century and on into the 21st century, as the limitations and unwanted side effects of mainstream medicine have become more and more evident, the public have shown a growing interest in more natural medicinal products, including essential oils, for therapeutic, cosmetic and aromatic benefit. The use of essential oils never ceased, but the scientific revolution minimized the popularity and use of essential oils in one's everyday life. Today's heightened awareness regarding the use of synthetics coupled with the increased availability of aromatherapy information within books and the Internet has refuelled the use of essential oils for therapeutic, cosmetic, fragrant and spiritual use.

The natural chemical composition of each essential oil differs according to the plant from which it is extracted and therefore the therapeutic benefits of each oil can also differ.

One thing all essential oils have in common is their ability to be readily absorbed by the skin. That's because their unique molecular structure allows them to pass through the cells that make up the outer, semi permeable layers of the skin and into the bloodstream and cells where they can have beneficial effects.

Here's an interesting experiment you might like to try to prove this to yourself. Garlic has been used medicinally for nearly 5000 years. Its unique anti-viral and anti-bacterial chemicals help treat high blood pressure, coughs, colds, acne and asthma.

Garlic oil also contains essential oils. Break open a capsule of the oil and massage it into your skin, somewhere on your body. Within a few hours you should be able to smell the garlic on your breath without ever having eaten it! That's because the oils have been absorbed through your skin and have made their way around your body to the respiratory system. Be careful - garlic oil has been known to irritate the skin in sensitive people.

Another thing all essential oils have in common is that they are to a lesser to greater extent, naturally anti-bacterial and antiseptic, so using a cream or lotion containing an essential oil will go some way to help keep spots and pimples at bay.

Essential oils are highly concentrated substances and should always be diluted in a vegetable-based carrier cream, lotion or oil before application to the skin. Sunflower and sweet almond oils are light and easy to use. If your skin is dry, heavier oils such as avocado or wheat germ may be more suitable. Most vegetable oils contain naturally occurring vitamins which are also of great benefit to the health and appearance of the skin.

Do not apply essential oils directly to the skin, dilute them according to the following guidelines:

20 drops of essential oil to 60 ml of carrier oil or lotion.
10 drops of essential oil to 30 ml of carrier oil or lotion.
5 drops of essential oil to 15 ml of carrier oil or lotion.

Please also note that you should use these oils for external use only and avoid contact with the eyes.

Do not use essential oils on babies or young children without the advice of a qualified aromatherapist. If you are epileptic, have liver damage, are taking medicines, have cancer, or have any other medical problem, consult qualified aromatherapist or your medical practitioner before using these blends.

A skin patch test should be conducted prior to using an essential oil that you've never used before. If you suffer an adverse reaction stop using the blend immediately.

The author cannot be held responsible for any adverse reactions experienced from using these home-made treatments and the reader uses them at his or her own risk. Consult your doctor or a qualified aromatherapist if in doubt.

Naturally Smooth Away Lines and Wrinkles and Rejuvenate Aging Skin

If you have frown lines, crows feet or lines at the corner of your mouth you know how depressing it can be to watch your face getting older in the mirror every morning. Let's face it, we all want to look as young as possible for as long as possible but may not want to resort the the surgeon's knife or paralyzing face injections.

Whether you like it or not, you live in a very superficial society where looks and appearance have a huge effect on all parts of your life, from sex and relationships to employment and social acceptance.

If you are 40 or over and you do nothing now, things are only going to get worse. If you let your face slowly degenerate into a tired-looking, wrinkly man, one day you will suddenly realize you look like your dad! Perhaps you've tried both conventional and alternative 'cures' anti-aging face creams before without much success and this has left you feeling let down and hopeless.

Thousands of years ago, in ancient Egypt, they believed that their divine Kings were destined, upon death, to undertake a long journey to the afterlife. To help them prepare for and survive this quest, the bodies of the dead were mummified or preserved so that they might arrive in the next world as fresh as a daisy.

Part of the preservation process was to cover the body in a natural oil that was renowned for it's 'death defying' effects on the skin. This treatment was so effective that, thousands of years later when modern archaeologists uncovered their graves, the skin of the long-since dead was still perfectly preserved! This precious, 'immortality oil' is still used today and is called frankincense.

Deeply Moisturize with Frankincense. Frankincense has been used as far back as ancient Egypt to preserve the skin. They used frankincense to mummify their dead, whose skin, thousands of years later, remains intact! As well as a skin preserver, it tones, smooths, moisturizes, restores dry skin and slows down the appearance of wrinkles.

Cleanse and Nourish with Neroli. Neroli is considered very nourishing for the skin and, like lavender, helps stimulate the growth of fresh, new, plump skin cells. This prevents dry skin from looking parched and tired. It also has mildly antiseptic properties.

Heal and Rejuvenate with Lavender. Lavender is a plant that has been used for centuries to rejuvenate and refresh tired-looking skin. It does so by stimulating the production of new, healthy skin cells.

Nourish and Restore with Carrot Seed. This essential oils restores tone and elasticity to mature skin that often tends to be try and inflexible. It is also known for it's ability to remove age spots, reduce wrinkles and improve the blood supply to the skin.

The Deep, Penetrating Moisture of Sandalwood. Sandalwood brings balance back to the skin. It is a natural antiseptic that softens and deeply moisturizes dry, mature or wrinkled skin.

The next two natural extracts are not essential oils but are known to be very beneficial skin treatments.

Rose Hip Seed Oil. Rose hip seed oil is extracted from the seeds of a rose bush called rosa moschata or rosa rubiginosa which grows wild in the southern Andes. It is unique among vegetable oils in containing retinol (vitamin A) in the form of retinoic acid which studies show reduces the appearance of wrinkles and brightens skin.

Rose hip oil also contains vitamin C and omega-6 and omega-3 essential fatty acids, known to heal scar tissue. It is used for a variety of skin conditions, including dermatitis, acne and eczema but it is in the field of anti-aging that rose hip oil is best 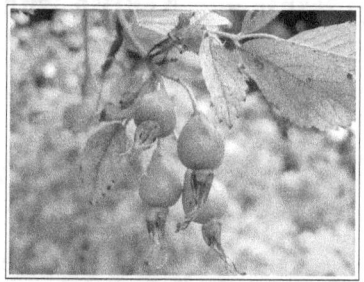 known because of it's ability to soften fine lines, fade irregular pigmentation and diminish the damage caused by sunlight.

Another key benefit is this oil's ability to be absorbed into the skin without leaving a greasy feel. This is because it is classed as a 'dry oil' so it penetrates to the deepest layers of the skin where it regenerates skin cells and encourages the protection of collagen and elastin, the skin's supportive proteins. This results in firmer, smoother, and more youthful skin with greater elasticity. Rosehip seed oil also contains a high amount of vitamin E, which further promotes healthy skin.

Other Anti-Aging Skin Treatments

Retinol

Retinol is a form of vitamin A that comes from animal sources such as cod liver oil, butter, margarine, liver, eggs, cheese, and milk.

When applied to the skin in a cream or lotion, retinol acts in a similar way to lavender essential oil by speeding up the rate at which new skin cells appear and the old ones fall away, so promoting a fresher appearance.

It also increases the production of collagen, the skin's supportive protein, to give a more youthful appearance and reduce fine lines.

Alpha Hydroxy Acid

Alpha hydroxy acids are natural and synthetic chemical compounds derived from food products such as sugar cane (glycolic acid), sour milk (lactic acid), apples (malic acid), citrus fruits (citric acid) and grape wine (tartaric acid).

They are well-known for their use in the cosmetics industry and are often found in products claiming to reduce wrinkles or the signs of aging. All these natural acids, to one degree or another, penetrate the epidermis or upper most layer of the skin to act as an exfoliator, that is, they encourage the shedding of old, dead skin cells that can make the skin look dull.

This allows new, fresh skin cells to come to the surface which in turn make the skin look fresher and smoother. In varying concentrations, these acids are also used to repair sun damage, skin discoloration and acne.

Sun Screen

One of the best and most basic ways to delay the signs of aging is to use a sunscreen. Sunscreen, sun block, sun lotion or sun cream is a lotion, spray, gel or other topical product that absorbs or reflects some of the sun's ultraviolet (UV) radiation on the skin exposed to sunlight and thus helps protect against sunburn.

Excessive exposure to direct sunlight is potentially harmful and, if you do not wear sun protective clothing or use suitable sunscreen, can result in sunburn and increased risk of skin aging and skin cancer.

Products with a higher SPF (Sun Protection Factor) level provide greater protection against ultraviolet radiation. Choose a broad-spectrum sunscreen that blocks both UVA and UVB rays and apply thickly enough to get the full SPF protection.

You should apply a sunscreen 15 to 30 minutes before exposure and 15 to 30 minutes after the sun exposure begins. You should re-apply the cream after activities such as swimming or sweating.

The sun's rays are strongest between 11 am and 3 pm so if you are outside during these times either apply a high protection level sunscreen and/or wear a hat with a brim, clothes that cover your arms and legs, and anti-UV sunglasses to protect against ultraviolet radiation entering the eyes.

A limited amount of unprotected exposure to the sun's rays is recommended because an over-use of sunscreen also interferes with vitamin D production, leading to possible deficiency.

Doctors recommend spending small amounts of time in the sun, for example, ten to fifteen minutes of sun exposure at least two times per week to the face, arms, hands or back, without sun protection to ensure adequate production of vitamin D. If you feel you are not getting enough exposure to therapeutic amounts of sun, a vitamin D supplement may be of benefit.

More Anti-Aging Skin Tips

Sleep Yourself Younger. To keep aging at bay get plenty of sleep. If you don't get 8 to 9 hours at night it can really show on the skin.

Fill Out Lines. Drink two liters of water a day. The internal hydration plumps your skin and fills out lines.

Fade Age Spots. To fade age spots dab lemon juice onto them morning and night. It works if you keep it doing it. Stop and the spots will darken again.

How to Solve Other Skin Problems Naturally

Oily and Greasy Skin

Here's a drug-free, alcohol-free, natural, gentle way to treat greasy and oily skin.

If you have oily or greasy skin you know how difficult it is to control without the use of harsh, skin-stripping alcohols or overly-drying soaps and detergents. Having skin that is excessively oily or greasy can make you very self-conscious. You worry about appearing 'shiny' or what someone will think if they touch your face.

If that wasn't enough, oil and grease is prone to clog your pores which then encourages the growth of bacteria and the appearance of spots and black heads. The last thing oily and greasy skin needs is a cream or lotion containing vegetable or mineral oils as these will only add to the problem. Try to find a light, non-perfumed, non-colored gel and add the following essential oils to it for a natural solution.

Spot-Busting, Grease-Cutting, Antiseptic Cypress. Cypress extract is naturally antiseptic, helping to first eliminate spots and blackheads. It's deep, penetrating properties will then cleanse deep down to stop them coming back. It is also a natural astringent, helping to naturally done the skin.

Balance and Heal with Geranium. Geranium has a balancing effect on the skin, restoring excessively dry skin to it's natural state by normalizing the secretion of sebum, the skin's own natural oil.

Detoxify with Juniper Berry. Juniper Berry is another naturally astringent and antiseptic extract that, together with Cypress, will help keep your skin clear of oil and grease, destroy spots and blemishes (and prevent them from coming back) and gently tone the skin.

Juniper Berry also has the unique ability to 'detoxify' the skin, gently flushing out impurities from the pores to give you a deep-down clean feeling. Please not that the skin may appear to get worse in the initial stages of use before it begins to improve as waste products are expelled from the skin. This is perfectly natural and temporary.

Dry Skin

If you have dry skin you know how upsetting and irritating this condition can be, especially if the problem is where your skin can be seen by others such as your face, arms or legs. Let's face it, dry and flaky skin is not attractive. It can sap your confidence and make you feel less attractive and more like hiding away from people's inquisitive stares.

Parched tight skin needs drenching in deep penetrating moisture to restore and heal. These oils have been used for hundreds of years to restore dry skin to it's normal, supple, comfortable state.

The Deep, Penetrating Moisture of Sandalwood. Sandalwood brings balance back to the skin. It penetrates deep down to soften and calm the irritation and itchiness that often accompanies dry skin.

Heal and Rejuvenate with Lavender. Lavender is a plant that has been used for centuries to heal and restore the skin. It is gently anti-bacterial, soothes eczema and stimulates the growth of fresh, healthy new skin cells.

Soothe, Calm and Moisturize with Clary Sage. Clary Sage is very soothing and helps to lock in moisture. It also has anti-inflammatory properties and so helps you to stop making dry skin worse by scratching.

Deeply Moisturise with Frankincense. Frankincense has been used as far back as ancient Egypt to preserve the skin. They used frankincense to mummify their dead, whose skin, thousands of years later, remains intact! As well as a skin preserver, it tones, smooths, moisturizes, restores dry skin and slows down the appearance of wrinkles.

Cleanse and Nourish with Neroli. Neroli is considered very nourishing for the skin and, like lavender, helps stimulate the growth of fresh, new, plump skin cells. This prevents dry skin from looking parched and tired. It also has mildly antiseptic properties.

Shaving Rash and Other Skin Irritations?

If you really want to enjoy your daily shave and if you want to stop worrying about whether your skin will or will not ruin your day, simply use these soothing, cooling natural oils.

Soothing and cooling natural relief from shaving rash, irritations and itchy skin. Shaving will once again be a pleasure with this cream. Ideal for soothing all kinds of unpleasant rashes. Oils of tea tree, chamomile and lavender will restore tranquillity and stop further irritation.

Heal and Cleanse with Tea Tree. Tree tree is one of the most popular essential oils in the world. It is well known for it's natural anti-bacterial and anti-septic properties making it an ideal healing balm for those accidental nicks and scratches. It also soothes and calms the skin, stopping irritation and inflammation before it starts.

Heal and Rejuvenate with Lavender. Lavender is a plant that has been used for centuries to heal and restore the skin. It is gently anti-bacterial, soothes the skin and stimulates the growth of fresh, healthy new skin cells to rapidly repair shaving damage.

Calm and Moisturize with Clary Sage. Clary Sage is very soothing and helps to lock in moisture. It also has anti-inflammatory properties and so helps you to stop making irritated and itchy skin worse by scratching.

Soothe and Cool with Chamomile. Chamomile extract is famous for it's soothing, calming and cooling properties. It is very good for sensitive and dry skin as it helps to relieve itchiness, redness and inflammation.

For more anti-aging tips go to goodallcopywriting.com and visit the blog.

Spots, Pimples, Boils, Blemishes and Acne

Say goodbye to those stubborn blemishes and stop them coming back with regular use of this cream. These powerful yet gentle antiseptic and anti-bacterial oils cleanse and deep clean the skin of impurities.

Heal and Cleanse with Tea Tree. Tree tree is one of the most popular essential oils in the world. It is well known for it's natural anti-bacterial and anti-septic properties making it an ideal destroyer of spot-causing skin bugs. It also soothes and calms the skin, stopping the irritation and inflammation often associated with acne.

Heal and Rejuvenate with Lavender. Lavender is a plant that has been used for centuries to heal, cleanse and clear the skin. It is gently anti-bacterial and soothing. It penetrates deeply to stimulate the growth of fresh, healthy new skin cells to replace those afflicted with blemishes.

Soothe, Calm and Moisturize with Clary Sage. Clary sage is very soothing and helps to lock in moisture. Moisturized skin heals more quickly.

It also has anti-inflammatory properties and so helps you to stop making spots and acne worse by scratching.

Bacteria Destroying, Pain Killing Eucalyptus. Eucalyptus is a very powerful and penetrating natural antiseptic and antibacterial extract. It will penetrate the skin deeply and clear, cleanse and heal from within.

Not only does it wipe out most types of spot-causing germs and bacteria, it also acts as a mild, natural local painkiller, so relieving you of the hurt and ache often associated with certain types of acne.

Balance and Heal with Geranium. Geranium has a balancing effect on the skin by normalizing the secretion of sebum, the skin's own natural oil. Excessive sebum production can block pores and make the skin oily which encourages the formation of spot-creating bacteria. It also acts as a natural skin toner and reduces inflammation. It's ability to naturally relieve acne is well documented.

Antiseptic, Astringent, Acne-clearing Cedarwood. Cedarwood is very antiseptic and mildly astringent, so helping to both cleanse and tone the skin. It is another natural extract that is well known as an effective treatment for acne.

Eczema & Psoriasis

Don't let eczema and psoriasis destroy your life. Avoid years of itching, scratching, pain and ugly skin with this a safe, plant-based skin treatment that contains a unique blend of natural ingredients known to reverse the effects of eczema and psoriasis and cure your skin condition forever.

Current medical treatments offer no cure and can also have side effects. If you go to your doctor he or she will more than likely prescribe a corticosteroids cream. Trouble is, prolonged use of topical corticosteroids is thought to increase the risk of side effects, the most common of which is the skin becoming thin and fragile.

In addition, high-strength steroids used over large areas may be significantly absorbed into the body, causing further health problems.

Over the years you've probably tried just about everything to relieve your eczema without much success, otherwise you wouldn't be reading this. You've probably tried to come to terms with your belief that you would have to suffer with and be self-conscious about, this distressing skin condition for the rest of your life. Don't despair, it doesn't have to be this way! There is another, all-natural, side-effect-free solution your doctor won't have told you about.

There's an amazing natural treatment that contains a powerful combination of natural ingredients (detailed below) that have been that have been used for centuries to deeply soothe heal, nourish and restore eczema and psoriasis-prone skin.

Heal and Rejuvenate with Lavender. Lavender is a plant that has been used for centuries to heal and restore the skin. It is gently anti-bacterial, soothes Eczema and stimulates the growth of fresh, healthy new skin cells.

Deeply Moisturise with Frankincense. Frankincense has been used as far back as ancient Egypt to preserve the skin. They used Frankincense to mummify their dead, whose skin, thousands of years later, remains intact! As well as a skin preserver, it tones, smooths, moisturizes, restores dry skin and slows down the appearance of wrinkles.

Sooth and Cool with Chamomile. Camomile extract is famous for it's soothing, calming and cooling properties. It is very good for sensitive and dry skin as it helps to relieve itchiness, redness and inflammation.

Nourish and Restore with Carrot Seed. This essential oils restores tone and elasticity to the skin and removes toxins. It has long been knows as an effective natural treatment for eczema and psoriasis.

Balance and Heal with Geranium. Geranium has a balancing effect on the skin, restoring excessively dry skin to it's natural state by normalising the secretion of sebum, the skin's own natural oil. Geranium also reduces inflammation and relieves dry eczema.

Coconut Oil. Coconut oil is extracted from the kernel or meat of matured coconut harvested from the coconut palm. Compared to other vegetable oils, coconut oil easily penetrates the skin to help keep it soft, smooth and to reduce inflammation. It also enhances the healing of wounds, blisters, rashes and eczema.

Coconut oil also reduces inflammation and redness of the skin,enhances the tissue healing and repair, maintains the natural chemical balance of the skin, softens the skin and helps to prevent flaking and dryness and protects to the skin from the damaging effects of ultraviolet rays.

Eliminate Eye Bags, Dark Circles and Wrinkles

The skin under your eyes is very thin at only 0.5mm thick. This is one of the reasons why normal aging processes of the skin are far more visible around our eyes.

There are two main kinds of baggy eyes: those caused by fluid retention and those caused by fat. As we age, the skin around your eyes loses its elasticity, and the connective tissue in the skin weakens, which can result in loose skin that forms folds in the eyelids.

The fat that cushions the eye sockets then moves forward, out of the eye sockets and accumulates in bulging bags around the eyelids.

Another reason for puffy eyes is eyelid oedema or the accumulation of water around the eye due to poor lymphatic circulation and increased capillary permeability.

The weakened skin folds more easily causing puffy baggy eyes and the veins beneath this tissue show through as dark circles. There are internal and external ways to keep your eyes looking fresh and reduce eye bags and dark circles.

Avoid drinking too much alcohol and eating salty foods.

Get a good night's sleep – at least 8-9 hours.

For a quick fix, fill the sink with ice cubes and cold water, then dunk your face in for 30 seconds or as long as you can stand it or place chilled tea bags or sliced cucumbers over your eyes.

Juice a cucumber and apply around the eyes for a cooling and soothing eye treat. Store excess in refrigerator for up to 10 days.

For puffy and swollen eyes, make a wet compress of 4 tablespoons of freshly grated raw potato. Place on the eyes for about 15 minutes and then rinse with cold water.

To reduce swelling and for bags under the eyes, brew a cup of strong rosehip tea. Soak 2 cotton balls in the tea or use 2 tea bags, lie down and place over the eyes.

Do not apply cream moisturizer around your eyes at bedtime. Instead use a gel-formula eye moisturizer, which will help firm and tighten the area and thereby reduce swelling.

Some people have found that reducing gluten and/or sugar in their diet reduces dark under eye circles.

A natural extract taken from sea plants also does the skin around the eyes a lot of good.

Algae extract, which comes from sea weed and pond scum, is rich in many different kinds of minerals, anti-oxidants, enzymes, amino acids and natural plant sugars, all of which have a beneficial effect on the delicate skin around the eyes. The natural sugars, alginates and enzymes in algae enable the skin to retain moisture more easily by binding water into the epidermis, which in turn keeps the skin soft and supple and helps reduce and prevent fine lines and wrinkles.

Other elements in this extract also act as a natural skin toner, not only firming up slack under eye skin to reduce the appearance of eye bags but also protecting collagen in the skin's from damage that can cause the eyes to look tired and old.

The extract also contains trace elements and nutrients that play a large part in maintaining good skin health and circulation such as copper, silicon, iron and zinc. Dark circles under the eyes are often attributed to poor circulation in that area, therefore using algae extract in combination with gentle massage may be of benefit.

Easy Home-Made Beauty Treatments

You don't have to spend hundreds on ready-made store products in order to have health-looking, soft, clear skin or shiny, sexy looking hair.

You can use commonplace products you probably already have in your kitchen or bathroom cabinet to achieve the exact same benefits but only spending a fraction of the money.

I selected the following home-made treatments because they are easy to make and the ingredients are cheap and readily available. They can be fun to make and even more fun to try on yourself or your partner.

Facial Treatments

If you are prone to acne breakouts, try this three step natural home-made treatment of scrub, face mask and moisturize and you should see an improvement without the need for the harsh chemicals you find in store-bought acne treatments.

Honey Cleansing Scrub

Mix together one tablespoon of honey, one tablespoon of finely ground almonds and half a teaspoon of lemon juice. Rub gently onto face. Rinse off with warm water.

Tomato Mask for Acne

Remove skin and seeds and mash quarter of a tomato, two teaspoon of plain yogurt, one teaspoon of mashed cucumber, two teaspoons of aloe gel, three teaspoons of oatmeal powder and two crushed mint leaves (crushed). Mix the ingredients together in a bowl and apply to the face and leave on for about 10 minutes. Rinse with warm water then moisturize with an oil-free lotion or cream.

Firming Face Mask

Whisk together one tablespoon honey, one egg white, one teaspoon glycerin and enough flour to form a paste. Smooth over face and throat. Leave on for 10 minutes and rinse off with warm water.

Rosewater Toner for Dry, Sensitive or Mature Skin

Mix together in a bottle three quarters of a cup of rosewater, 6 drops of glycerin and two thirds of a cup of witch hazel. Use as a normal toner by applying all over the face with a cotton wool pad.

Honey and Almond Scrub

Skin always looks brighter and smoother when it has been ex-exfoliated. Try this natural scrub.

Mix in a blender 2 tablespoons of slivered almonds or buy read-made crushed almonds. Put these in a bowl and add half a small jar of cold cream and one tablespoon of honey. Smooth the mixture onto the face in a circular motion for up to two minutes and rinse off.

All Over Body Exfoliator

Mix an eighth of a cup of olive oil with one heaped tablespoon of sea salt and scrub all over in the shower. Rinse off and pat dry with a towel.

Flaky Face Scrub

Mix a quarter of a cup of honey with a quarter of a teaspoon of ground cloves and smooth over your face. Leave on 15 minutes then rinse thoroughly.

Gentle Skin Exfoliator

Mix three teaspoons of fine oatmeal with three teaspoons of double or heavy cream. Apply to your skin and rub lightly then rinse off.

Soothing Skin Toner for Wrinkles

Mix together two tablespoons of vodka, one tablespoon of fennel seeds and one and a half teaspoons of honey. Let this sit for three days then strain through a sieve to remove the seeds. Apply to the face with a cotton pad as a toner. Mixture can be diluted to suit.

Avocado Honey Mask

Peel and slice one avocado and puree with one tablespoon of honey. Pat mixture onto the face until the mast feels extremely tacky to the touch. Leave on for up to 30 minutes and then rinse with warm water.

Apricot-Walnut Scrub For Normal to Dry Skin

Mix together the pulp of one mashed apricot, 1 teaspoon of rolled oats, one teaspoon of ground walnut shells, one teaspoon of witch hazel and half a teaspoon of safflower oil. Apply to the face and let it set for 10 minutes and then rinse off.

Brewer's Yeast Face Mask for Dry Skin

Mix together quarter of a cup of yeast powder (you should find it in the baking section of your local supermarket) with one tablespoon of water to form a soft paste. Then stir in one tablespoon of wheatgerm oil and one egg yolk. Smooth over your face and let it sit on your skin for up to five minutes then rinse thoroughly. Now apply your usual moisturizer.

Firming Face Mask for Dry Skin

Whisk together one tablespoon of honey, one egg white, one teaspoon of glycerin (glycerin can be found at your drug store) and enough flour to form a paste.

Smooth over face and throat and leave on for 10 minutes then rinse off with warm water.

Moisture Mask for Dry Skin

Mix two tablespoons of honey with two teaspoons of milk. Smooth over face and throat and leave on for 10 minutes then rinse off with warm water.

Smoothing Skin Lotion for Dry Skin

Mix one teaspoon of honey with with one teaspoon of vegetable oil and a quarter teaspoon of lemon. Rub into your hands, elbows, heels and anywhere that feels dry.
Leave on 10 minutes then rinse. off with water.

Get Healthy Glowing Skin Naturally for Dry Skin

This recipe will help tighten your pores and make your face glow.

Mix together one teaspoon of honey, one teaspoon of cold milk and one or two drops of lemon juice. Apply to your face and leave on for 15 minutes and then rinse off with cold water.

Apple Sauce Face Mask for Oily Skin

Slice one apple and cook in water until it can be mashed. Add one teaspoon of lemon juice and one teaspoon of dried herb such as parsley, sage, rosemary or whatever you've got in the cupboard. Apply to the face and leave for five minutes then rinse with warm water and apply your usual moisturizer.

Carrot Face Mask for Oily Skin

Mix together one tablespoon of carrot juice, one tablespoon of honey, 10 drops of lemon juice and one tablespoon of flour. Mix the ingredients into a paste and apply to your face for 20 minutes then wash off.

Cucumber Mask for Oily Skin

Put half of a cucumber into a blender and blend until smooth. Apply mixture to your face and leave on for 15 minutes then rinse.

Lemon Juice Toner for Oily Skin

This toner will reduce shine. Combine 10 drops of lemon juice with half a cup of cold water. Saturate a cotton pad with the mixture and dab over skin. Do not rinse.

Apple & Honey Mask for Oily or Acne Prone Skin

Grate one medium sized apple and mix with five tablespoons of honey. Smooth over your skin and let sit for 10 minutes then rinse off with cool water.

Blemished Skin Mask

Mix together one ripe, shopped tomato with one teaspoon of lemon juice and one tablespoon of instant oatmeal or rolled oats. Blend everything until just combined. Apply to the skin, making sure the mixture is thick enough to stay on the blemished areas. If necessary add a little more oatmeal to thicken the mask, and then scrub it off with a washcloth dipped in warm water.

Carrot Mask For Oily Skin

Boil three large carrots and mash them or mix in a food processor. Add five tablespoons of honey or yogurt and apply to the skin. Leave on for 15-20 minutes then rinse with warm water.

Cucumber Yogurt Facial For Normal/Oily Skin

Puree half a cucumber in a blender and mix in one tablespoon of plain yogurt. Apply to your face and leave for up to 30 minutes and then rinse well.

Facial Scrub for Acne

Blend in a food processor two cups of powdered oatmeal and one small pack of blanched almonds. Mix this powder with one small bar of grated baby soap. Use about one teaspoon to scrub your face or two to three teaspoons for a body scrub. Store in a tightly sealed jar.

Strawberries and Cream Astringent for Oily or Blemished Skin

Mash one handful of strawberries and add one tablespoon of heavy cream. Mix well and spread thickly on the face and neck and let it sit on your skin for 10 minutes. Remove with a tissue and splash face with cool water.

Strawberry Mask

Mix in a blender half a cup of natural yogurt, three chopped strawberries and half a cup of oats. Put the mask on your face with your fingers and lie back and relax for 15 minutes then rinse off with warm water. And for an extra boost put slices of cucumber on your eyes.

Egg Yolk Mask

A good mask for tightening up pores. Take one beaten egg and apply liberally to the face with a cotton pad or ball and leave for 15 minutes then rinse off with cool water.

Honey Oatmeal Mask for Oily Skin

Just mix honey and oatmeal into a paste and apply to your face for 15 minutes. The oatmeal will absorb the excess oil off your skin. Rinse with warm water.

Natural Help for Dandruff

Instead of spending money on store-bought anti-dandruff shampoos full of chemicals, why not give these methods a try first?

Method 1. Mix one part of antiseptic mouthwash with 9 parts of water and massage to scalp. Rinse after 10 minutes.
Method 2. Mix 3 tbsp of lime juice with ¼ cup coconut oil and massage to scalp. Shampoo after 1 hour.

Method 3. Boil oat meal and massage to scalp, comb after 10 minutes and shampoo after 15 minutes. Repeat this once in week.

Sex-Up Bath Time

There's nothing quite like taking a long, hot, relaxing soak in the bath, especially if it's with a special someone. It's even better if you know the bubble bath is doing your skin good too, so get out the candles, take the phone off the hook, put on the romantic music and try these skin-soothing, easy-to-make home-made bath additives.

Foaming Vanilla Honey Bath

Mix together one cup of sweet almond oil or other light vegetable oils such as olive or sesame, half a cup of honey, half a cup of store-bought liquid soap and one tablespoon of vanilla extract. Pour half a cup of the mixture under running water into the tub. Relax and enjoy! Put the remainder in an air-tight container for later use and refrigerate for up-to 30 days.

Home Made Milk and Sea Salt Bath

This milk bath is great for all skin types. Into a large bowl place one cup of instant, dried skimmed milk powder and add three quarters of a cup of fine or coarse sea salt and mix well. Remove half the mixture and place in a small bowl and add to this 20-25 15-20 crops of essential oil. See the skincare section for oils that are great for the skin. Stir the mixture well. Add this back into the main bowl and mix thoroughly.

Store your milk bath in a glass jar with a tight fitting lid. Scoop out about a third of a cup and dissolve under running bath water. This recipe makes enough for about 5 or 6 baths.

Honey Milk Bath

Mix together in a bowl one cup of honey, 2 cups of milk, one cup of salt and a quarter of a cup of baking soda. Fill the bath and pour the mixture into the water. Then add about half a cup of baby oil and essential oils or fragrance of your choice.

The Super Soaker

Add one quart of whole milk and three tablespoons of lemon juice to a very warm bath. Slice some lemon and put in the water too. Soak for at least 15 minutes for silky smooth skin.

Feet

If you've been on your feet all day or just want to soften the skin, here's a home made bath soak.

Milk Bath For Your Feet

Warm 3 cups whole milk in a saucepan. In another bowl mix half a cup of coarse salt and a third of a cup of olive oil. Soak your feet in the milk for 10 minutes then rinse. Scrub your feet with a salt and oil mixture then rinse and apply a moisturizer. Put on some thick sock to seal in the softness.

Smoothing Foot Exfoliant

Mix together eight 8 strawberries, two tablespoons of olive oil, one teaspoon of salt and one teaspoon of finely chopped almonds.

Massage all over feet rinse off and dry thoroughly.

Banana Foot Cream

If you get dry feet, try this overnight moisturizer. Mix together half a mashed banana, one tablespoon of honey, juice from half a lemon and one tablespoon of margarine. Smear on your feet and wear thick socks to bed. Wash off in the morning.

Massage Oils

There's nothing sexier than getting a nice massage from your special friend, so here are some simple and easy massage oil blends to put you in the mood. If you don't have anyone to massage you, these make great moisturizing body oils for smooth, supple and healthy skin.

You will need to source the essential oils either on-line or from your local health food shop. Good base oils are almond, wheatgerm, apricot, grape seed, sunflower and olive oil. Mix your blend either in a small glass or plastic screw top bottle. Shake the bottle well before using.

Erotic Massage Oil

Coriander 3 drops, Frankincense 3 drops, Lime 2 drops, Rose 2 drops. Add to 1 oz base oil.

Sandalwood Massage Oil

Eight to 10 teaspoons of grape seed oil, six drops sandalwood oil, two drops lavender oil, two drops rosewood oil and two drops rose oil.

Forest Nights Massage Oil

10 teaspoons of grape seed oil, 5 drops rosewood oil, 2 drops cedar wood oil and 2 drops chamomile oil.

Manly Massage Oil

Quarter of a cup of mineral/baby oil, eighth of a cup of castor oil, eighth of a cup of sweet almond oil, six drops of sandalwood oil, four drops of bay oil, three 3 drops of bergamot oil, two drops of lime oil.

Sexual Energy Oil

Two drops of cardamom oil, four drop of ginger oil, five drops of patchouli oil and four drops of sandalwood oil. Mix into half an ounce of carrier oil.

For more anti-aging tips go to goodallcopywriting.com and visit the blog.

Hair Care

Dry Hair Conditioner

You will need one 1 ounce of fresh rosemary or a few drops of rosemary essential oil, one pint of hot water and one egg. Steep the rosemary in the water for 20 minutes (if using the fresh plant). Cool. Beat in the egg. Add a few drops of rosemary essential oil if using. Massage into the hair and rinse.

Split Ends Treatment

Hot Oil Treatment

Half a cup of olive oil, half a cup of boiling water and the liquid from four vitamin E capsules. Simply poke a hole in the vitamin E capsules with a pin and squeeze the liquid out. Place the olive oil, vitamin E liquid and boiling water into a large glass bottle or jar with a lid. Wrap a towel around the bottle to avoid burning yourself. Shake very well until the oil is emulsified. Then thoroughly massage into hair, taking care not to burn your head.

Wrap a plastic bag over your hair and wrap your head in hot towel that has been soaked in hot water then wrung out. Leave mixture on your hair for 30 minutes or overnight if your hair is more damaged, then shampoo as usual.

Deep Conditioner

One small jar of real mayonnaise and half of an avocado. In a medium sized bowl smash mayonnaise and avocado together with a fork until it's mixed together thoroughly. Smooth into hair all the way to the tips. Put on a shower cap and eave on for 20 minutes.

Hair Conditioner

Half a cup of honey and a quarter of a cup of olive oil. Use two tablespoons of oil for normal hair. Work a small amount at a time through your hair until coated. Cover hair with a shower cap and leave on 30 minutes. Remove the shower cap, shampoo well and rinse. Dry as normal.

Shine Boosting Hair Mask

Mash an over-ripe banana and combine with three drops of almond oil. Massage into dry hair, leave on for 15 minutes and then shampoo out.

Lemon and Aloe Vera Shampoo for Oily Hair

Two teaspoons of aloe vera gel (available at your local health food store and one tablespoon of lemon juice. Blend the ingredients together with a quarter of a cup of your regular hair shampoo. Wash hair then rinse well.

Egg Protein Shampoo

One egg, one teaspoon of olive oil, one teaspoon of lemon juice, one tablespoon of castile soap, half a cup of water or herbal tea and five drops of an essential oil of your choice.

Combine all the ingredients in a blender and whip until smooth. Shampoo with mixture using warm water. Store any remaining shampoo in the refrigerator for use the next day.

Frizzy Hair Treatment

One cup of water, half a cup of vinegar and half a cup of oatmeal water. To make oatmeal water, soak the oatmeal in hot water and leave it for two to three days at room temperature and then remove the oatmeal flakes with the use of cheesecloth or strainer. Rinse your hair with this mixture to help keep frizzy hair away.

Hot Oil Treatment for Dandruff

All you need is half a cup olive oil and half a cup boiling water. Pour the olive oil and boiling water into large glass bottle or jar with a lid. You may need to wrap a towel around the bottle to avoid burning yourself. Shake very well until the oil is emulsified.

Massage into hair, taking care not to burn your head. Put a shower cap or plastic bag over your hair and wrap your head in a hot towel that has been soaked in hot water then wrung out.

Leave mixture on your hair for half an hour then shampoo as usual.

Enhance Your Blond Hair Naturally

Chamomile is a natural hair lightener. Brew some chamomile tea and let cool completely then our on dry hair and leave on for 20 minutes then rinse or use the tea as a rinse after you shampoo. Alternatively, rinse hair with a solution of one tablespoon of lemon juice to one gallon of water after shampooing.

Cover or Enhance Grey

Before you reach for that bottle of hair chemical hair dry, try these natural solutions.

Boil potato peels in water, strain and cool. Use the strained water as an after-shampoo rinse to darken grey hair.

Sage covers the grey when used consistently over a period of time. Simmer half a cup of dried sage (find it in the herb and spice section of your local supermarket) in two cups of water for 30 minutes. Steep for 2-3 hours then strain and use as a rinse on clean hair. Leave it n until hair has dried and then rinse out.

Another dried herb you can try is rosemary. Mix one ounce of sage and one ounce of rosemary and one pint of water. Simmer for 30 minutes and strain. Massage into the scalp and the grey hair.

Another treatment is to mix 1 tablespoon of apple-cider vinegar with one gallon of warm water, use as final rinse.

Enrich Your Dark Hair Color Naturally

Brew one strong cup of espresso coffee and let it cool completely. Pour on dry hair and leave on for 20 minutes then rinse.

Cook an unpeeled potato in boiling water. Cool slightly and dip a pastry brush, cotton ball or cotton pad in the water, cover and saturate hair, being careful not to get any on your skin. Leave on hair for 20 minutes then rinse out.

Make a strong infusion of either rosemary, sage, raspberry leaves, parsley, black coffee or black tea then use as a rinse.

Enrich Your Red Hair Color Naturally

Use strong black coffee, rosehip tea or hibiscus tea as a final rinse.

Cucumber- Yogurt Eye Smoother and Moisturizer

This mixture will help to reduce puffiness and moisturize your eyes as well. The mixture must be made fresh for each use. Mix half a cup of chopped, skinned cucumber, a quarter of a cup of plain yogurt and one egg. Mix all of the ingredients until smooth, and apply mixture to closed eyes, covering the entire area surrounding the eyes. Apply a warm cloth over your eyes for 20 minutes then rinse your face with warm water.

The Anti-Aging Power of Antioxidants

Diet plays an important role in keeping mind and body young, healthy and sexy. There is a lot you can do to slow down the natural aging of cells and ward off common ailments.

A diet rich in antioxidants is a natural, simple way to keep your skin and body in the best possible condition but what exactly is an antioxidant?

Thousands of chemical reactions occur in our bodies every minute of every day. Without them our bodies would not be able to function properly. Many are the bi-product of breathing in of oxygen and the digestion of chemicals in our food and drink.

Whenever we are exposed to environmental pollution, drink alcohol, smoke, exercise, are exposed to the sun or take certain drugs, our bodies produce molecules called 'free radicals'. These are unstable molecules that carry a negative electrical charge in the form of a spare electron.

They try to rid themselves of this unwanted molecular 'baggage' by colliding with other molecules or they try to steal a positive charge from other molecules to neutralize their spare negative electron. This chemical offloading and stealing is known as oxidation. An excess of these free radicals can start chain reactions that damage cells, proteins, fats and genetic material in our bodies.

This damage has been linked to many health problems and diseases including hardening and furring up of the arteries, coronary heart disease, cataracts, arthritis, cancer and premature aging of the skin.

An antioxidant is a protective substance that helps to neutralize this damaging oxidation. They work by mopping up the negative charges on free radicals before they can trigger a damaging chain reaction. Antioxidants are found in varying amounts in foods such as vegetables, fruits, grain cereals, eggs, meat, legumes and nuts.

Although a normal diet high in antioxidants is good, experts agree that food alone cannot supply the optimum amounts needed to be effective – you would need to eat huge amounts of foods containing antioxidants for them to be effective and some antioxidants can be destroyed by storage and cooking.

Because the amount of antioxidants in any one food type can vary so much, if you are serious about maintaining your health and warding off age-related disease, taking supplements is well worth considering.

There follows a list of known antioxidants you should try to incorporate into your diet. You will find supplements for most of these age-fighters at your local health food shop or drug store. If you wish to purchase them over the Internet, which is usually cheaper and more convenient, go to the resources section at the end of this book for good places to buy.

Vitamin A and Beta-Carotene

Vitamin A is a fat soluble antioxidant that comes in two forms – retinol which is found in animal products like meat and milk, and carotenoids which come from fruits and vegetables. Both these forms are converted into vitamin A in the body.

The importance of vitamin A in skin health comes from its ability to treat severe forms of acne and psoriasis and repair sun damage and wrinkles. In recognition of this ability, the cosmetics industry has not been slow in including retinol in many anti-aging products.

Vitamin A is such a powerful antioxidant that several studies have suggested that dietary intake is important in reducing the risk of many cancers, including skin cancer. Dietary sources of vitamin A include halibut liver oil, liver, margarine, butter, cheese and eggs.

If vitamin A supplements are used, they are best limited to no more than 1500 mcg a day although intakes of up to 3000 mcg are considered safe.

Vitamin C

Vitamin C is a water soluble vitamin that cannot be produced in the human body and so has to be obtained from food and supplements on a daily basis. It plays an important role in the health and appearance of the skin because it promotes and maintains the production of elastin and collagen. Elastin and collagen fibers form up to seventy percent of the skin's structure and help to keep it smooth and supple.

Excessive exposure to sunlight produces free radicals that damage the skin's structure and cause wrinkles, dryness, thickening, dis-coloration and 'photo-aging'. Vitamin C has been shown to protect against damage caused by UV exposure by neutralizing these free radicals and promoting the production of new collagen.

The best food sources for vitamin C are, acerola cherry juice, camu pulp, rosehip syrup, blackcurrants, guavas, parsley and kale.

A good basic amount of vitamin C per day is 100-250 mg, however, research suggests that a higher intake of between 1000-3000 mg per day is preferable for optimum health. Such a large amount cannot normally be obtained from food alone, therefore a supplement is recommended for best results.

Vitamin E

Vitamin E is the collective name for a set of eight related tocopherols and tocotrienols, which are fat-soluble vitamins with antioxidant properties. Vitamin E is a preservative and protects the body's fats and cell membranes from free radical damage.

As far as skin health is concerned, vitamin E improves skin suppleness and its ability to heal, hence is present in many skin creams, both as a preservative for the cream's ingredients and for its benefits to the skin.

Dietary sources of vitamin E include, wheatgerm oil, soy bean oil, maize oil, safflower oil, sunflower oil and peanut oil.

A normal daily dosage of vitamin E is 10-1000 mg a day. High intakes of more than 3000 mg a day can be toxic.

Selenium

Selenium is an essential trace mineral needed for normal cell growth, hormone production and a healthy immune system. An adequate intake of selenium has been show to protect against many diseases such as cancer, arthritis, heart attack, infertility, stroke and emphysema.

In skin health, selenium, like vitamin A and E, has been shown to protect the skin against the damaging effects of UV radiation. A lack of this mineral has also been linked with psoriasis, age spots and wrinkling of the skin.

Good sources of selenium include Brazil nuts, whole grains, mushrooms, onions, garlic and broccoli. Suggested daily intake of Selenium is 100-200 mcg a day.

Riboflavin/Vitamin B2

Vitamin B2 plays an important role in the body's processing of proteins, fats and carbohydrates. It also plays a part in the production of hormones and red blood cells as well as helping to keep the skin, hair and eyes healthy. A lack in the diet can lead to a skin rash similar to eczema on the face and nose.

Riboflavin helps to protect the eye lens from attack by free radicals. In a study, subjects taking a B2 supplement nearly halved their risk of developing cataracts than those who did not take them.

Vitamin B2 is a water soluble vitamin that cannot be stored in the body, therefore a regular intake from the diet or supplement is essential for health. Good food sources include yeast extract, whole grains, eggs, dairy products, green leafy vegetables, pulses, wheat bran and soy flour;

Normal daily requirements are 1.6 mg per day but physically active people and those with a specific deficiency problem can take between 200-400 mg daily.

Copper

Although not an antioxidant itself, the presence of copper in the body is vital for the actions of other enzymes and vitamins involved in antioxidant activity. It is essential for the function of enzymes involved in antioxidant protection and helps with vitamin C absorption and the production of collagen, a structural protein that supports the skin and keeps it supple and healthy.

Good dietary sources of copper include, brewer's yeast, olives, nuts, pulses, cereals, wholemeal bread and dried fruit.

Despite many dietary sources, in general, around 50% of people get less than the recommended 0.8-3 mg recommended daily intake, therefore taking a supplement may be of benefit.

Manganese

Manganese is an antioxidant mineral that, along with vitamin C, is essential for the production of collagen, the substance that supports your skin and keeps is supple and healthy. Deficiency symptoms include scaly skin and poor growth of hair.

Good dietary sources include cereals, wholemeal bread, nuts, pulses, fruit, green leafy vegetables and black tea.

We lose manganese from the body every time we have a bowel motion, therefore a daily intake of up to 5 mg is recommended.

Zinc

An adequate intake of zinc is vital for sexual health in men both in terms of fertility and the health of the prostate gland but when looking particularly at skin health, we find that a lack of zinc in the diet can lead to eczema, psoriasis, acne and poor hair and nail growth.

Good dietary sources of zinc include brewer's yeast, hard cheese, wholemeal bread, eggs, pulses, wholegrain cereals, rice, green leafy vegetables and potatoes.

As with all the antioxidants mentioned in this book, obtaining enough to be therapeutic (15-30 mg a day) can be difficult from the diet alone and therefore supplementation may be beneficial.

Please note that doses of more than 30 mg daily should not be taken except under medical supervision or the advice of a dietitian.

Green Tea

Green and black tea both come from from the camellia sinesis shrub but green tea contains higher levels of an antioxidant known as a bioflavonoid.

Flavonoids are known to be far stronger antioxidants than either vitamin C or vitamin E and prevent cholesterol from blocking up the arteries.

People who regularly drink green tea have a lower risk of heart disease, stroke and high blood pressure.

They are also thought to prevent several types of cancer due to the presence of epigallocatechin gallate – a powerful anti-cancer compound.

Of particular interest is green tea's ability to protect against premature aging, a fact seized by cosmetic manufacturers who now include extracts in a wide variety of skin creams and lotions.

Drinking four cups of green tea daily is recommended but if you dislike the taste, it can also be taken as a supplement.

Co-enzyme Q10

Also known as ubiquinone, co-enzyme Q10 is a vitamin-like substance that works with vitamin E to form an antioxidant that protects against the hardening and furring up of the arteries and reduces the risk of heart disease.

Co-enzyme Q10 is present in all the body's cells where it is needed to generate energy from food and protects cells from disease and damage.

Cosmetics manufacturers have recognized its protective properties and added Q10 to skin care products to help reduce and prevent premature wrinkles and damage from sunlight.

A good dietary source of Q10 is yeast but for the optimal daily dose of 10-100 mg (300-600 mg for the treatment of specific illnesses) a supplement is recommended.

Pine Bark Extract

This extract comes from the bark of the French maritime pine tree. It contains proanthocyanidins - strong antioxidants that play a role in the stabilization of collagen and maintenance of elastin — proteins in connective tissue that support organs, joints, blood vessels, muscle and skin.

Proanthocyanidins antioxidants are 20 times more powerful than vitamin C and 50 times more potent than vitamin E and help strengthen all the blood vessels and improve the delivery of oxygen to the cells.

This extract also enhances the effectiveness of these vitamins and co-enzyme Q10 to create a powerful protective cocktail that reduces the risk of heart disease and stroke, improves circulation and strengthens blood vessels.

It's ability to thin the blood and prevent clotting make it a good alternative to aspirin that can be taken prior to any long-haul economy class flight to help reduce the risk of deep vein thrombosis. You can take 50-200 mg a day.

Cat's Claw

Cat's Claw is a vine native to South America where indigenous people have used the plant for medicinal purposes for over two thousand years. It gets its name name from hook-like thorns that resemble the claws of a cat. It contains potent antioxidants that protect against damage caused by sun exposure and smoking.

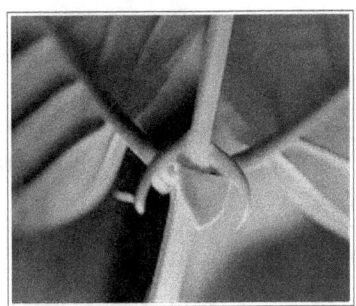

The alkaloids found in this plant have also been shown to be effective in the treatment of a wide range of ailments including Crohn's disease, gastric ulcers and tumors, parasites, colitis, gastritis, arthritis, rheumatism, diabetes, PMS, chronic fatigue syndrome, HIV, Alzheimer's disease, prostate conditions and in the treatment of AIDS in combination with AZT.

Ginkgo

Loss of memory and an increase in the experience of cold hands and feet are often seen as a sign of aging, but your circulation can be kept as healthy and efficient as possible, both through moderate regular exercise, and by taking herbs known to boost blood transmission to the brain, hands, feet and genitals.

Extract of ginkgo biloba contains unique chemicals called gingkolides and bilobalides, that not only offer protection against oxidative cell damage from free radicals, but are also known to relax blood vessels and increase blood flow to the hands and feet.

It also helps blood flow to the genitals, where it acts to strengthen and maintain an erection. In a study, half the participating males with erectile dysfunction enjoyed a return to full potency after six months of taking ginkgo. As well as boosting blood flow to the brain to improve memory, clinical trials have shown.

Ginkgo can also be ineffective in treating other age-related problems such as dementia and Alzheimer's Disease. Taking a minimum of 120 mg of ginkgo a day should be enough to notice benefits although these may not be noticeable until ten days to 12 weeks after use.

Bilberry

The bilberry comes from a small shrub found in Europe, Asia and North America. The dark purple fruit is smaller than that of the blueberry but with a fuller taste.

Bilberries contain anthocyanins, tannins and flavonoid glycosides - antioxidants that have been shown to combat many age-related eye disorders such as macular degeneration, cataracts, night blindness and glaucoma.

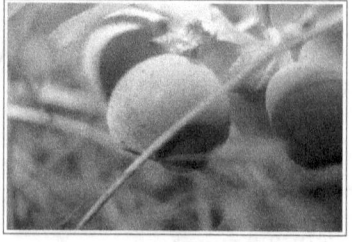

The antioxidants in bilberry protect light sensitive cells found in the eye and improves blood flow to the retina. Users have reported an improvement in their eyesight after only 15 days of use.

In one study, participants who had cataracts were given a combination of bilberry and Vitamin E. In all but three percent of cases, the deterioration in their eyesight was halted.

If you want to eat the fresh fruit, 20-60 grammes a day is recommended, alternatively, 80-160 mg of dry extract up to three times a day can be taken.

Red Grapeseed Extract

Red grape seed extract contains powerful antioxidants called proanthocyanidins that have been shown to treat heart disease, high blood pressure and high cholesterol.

This is because they protect the blood vessels from free radical damage, thin the blood and reduce the hardening and furring up of the arteries.

Because of its positive effect on the circulation, other diseases associated with poor blood flow such as diabetes, impotence, varicose veins, macular degeneration and thread veins can also be improved with this extract.

Grape seed extract may have other possible anti-disease properties, including accelerated wound healing, the reduction of skin cancer tumors and protection from ultra violet light damage to the skin.

Olive Oil

Olive oil is an oil obtained from the olive tree olea europaea, a traditional tree of the Mediterranean area and has been in use by man since 2,500 BCE. Today it is commonly used in cooking, cosmetics, pharmaceuticals and soaps. Olive oil contains potent antioxidants not found in other vegetable oils that give extra-virgin unprocessed olive oil its bitter and pungent taste.

Hydroxytyrosol is thought to be the main antioxidant in olives, and plays a significant role in the many health benefits attributed to this oil, including a protective effect against certain malignant tumors in the breast, prostate and digestive tract.

Olive oil is considerably rich in a mono-unsaturated fat called oleic acid. Studies suggest that a higher proportion of mono-unsaturated fats in the diet is linked with a reduction in the risk of coronary heart disease.

To achieve this possible benefit, olive oil should replace a similar amount of saturated fat found in meat and dairy products and not increase the total number of calories you eat in a day. There is a large body of clinical data to show that consumption of olive oil can also have favorable effects on cholesterol regulation because it controls the 'bad' levels of LDL cholesterol and raises levels of the 'good' HDL cholesterol,

In addition to the internal health benefits of olive oil, extra virgin olive oil has been known for generations, not only for its healing qualities, but also as a natural, deep penetration moisturizer with a reputation for regenerating and softening the skin.

Studies on mice showed that the application of olive oil immediately following exposure to UVB rays has a preventive effect on the formation of tumors and skin cancer.

Wolfberry or Goji Berry

The Wolfberry is a deciduous woody perennial plant native to south-eastern Europe and Asia, particularly China where it has long been used in traditional Chinese medicine.

The berries of this plant have come to be known as a 'superfood' due to their very high nutritional and antioxidant content including:

- 11 essential and 22 trace dietary minerals;
- 18 amino acids;
- 6 essential vitamins;
- 8 polysaccharides and 6 monosaccharides;
- 5 unsaturated fatty acids, including the essential fatty; acids, linoleic acid and alpha-linolenic acid;
- beta-sitosterol and other phytosterols;
- 5 carotenoids, including beta-carotene and zeaxanthin.

100 grams of dried berries can provide calcium, potassium, iron, zinc, selenium, riboflavin, vitamin C and beta-carotene.

Published studies have shown beneficial effects on cardiovascular and inflammatory diseases, vision-related diseases such as age-related macular degeneration and glaucoma and anti-cancer properties.

For more anti-aging tips go to goodallcopywriting.com and visit the blog.

Simple Anti-Aging Diet Changes That Can Prolong Life, Improve Health and Make You Look Younger

There is now a huge and growing body of evidence to show that a well-balanced 100% plant-based diet is the ideal vehicle for the promotion of human health. Based on whole grains, pulses, fruits, vegetables, seeds and nuts, it is these foods that provide all the essential nutrients – vitamins, minerals, essential fats, protein, starchy carbohydrate and fiber – that we must take into our bodies if we want not just to survive, but to thrive!

The Trouble With Too Much Protein

The problem with protein in the Western diet is actually more to do with eating too much than eating too little. Excessive protein consumption can lead to a number of serious health problems.

Studies show that vegan diets provide sufficient amounts of protein, automatically met by a balanced, varied diet including grains (e.g. rice) and pulses (e.g. beans).

Osteoporosis

Most of our body's calcium is in our bones. The small amount in our bloodstream plays an important role in functions such as muscle contraction and maintenance of the heartbeat.

Bloodstream calcium is constantly being lost through urine, sweat and feces. Replacement comes from the bones, which depend on fresh supplies from the food we eat.

Diets rich in animal protein, such as that found in cow's milk, make the blood more acidic. The body tries to neutralize this by drawing calcium from the bones into the bloodstream, which is filtered through the kidneys and lost through urine.

The more dairy consumed, the more calcium the body needs to balance the losses. Therefore too much protein actually leaches calcium from the bones and contributes to weak bones and osteoporosis. Countries whose populations eat low-protein diets have lower rates of osteoporosis and hip fractures.

Kidney Disease And Kidney Stones

Excess protein consumption produces more nitrogen than the body requires. This strains the kidneys, which must expel the extra nitrogen through urine, causing reduced kidney function.

Over time, individuals who consume very large amounts of animal protein, risk permanent loss of kidney function.

High animal protein diets also lead to more uric acid in the urine, and a general increase in urine acidity. Because of the acidity, the uric acid does not easily dissolve and can form into kidney stones.

Heart Disease And Stroke

Saturated animal fats found in meat and dairy products raise cholesterol and can increase the risk of heart disease and strokes by blocking blood flow through the arteries. If the blood flow to the heart is blocked, a heart attack can occur. If the blood flow to the brain is blocked, a stroke can occur.

Official dietary guidelines across the world recommend that no more than 10% of calories should come from saturated fats. In the UK, dairy foods contribute about 20% of total fat intake and over a third of saturated fat. Cholesterol is found only in animal products. Meat, fish, poultry, dairy products, and eggs all contain cholesterol, while plant products do not.

Choosing lean cuts of meat is not enough; the cholesterol is mainly in the lean portion. Many people are surprised to learn that chicken contains as much cholesterol as beef.

A diet rich in whole grains, vegetables, beans and fruits, is free of artery-clogging cholesterol and low in saturated fat.

Cancer

Too much fat in the diet is the food-related factor most often identified for increasing the risk of contracting cancer, but protein also plays a role.

Populations that eat meat and dairy products regularly are at an increased risk from cancers such as colon, breast, ovarian and prostate.

Cow's milk contains a powerful growth hormone – IGF-1 – that stimulates the growth of malignant cells and has been identified as a key factor in the growth of human cancer. People drinking milk have increased levels of IGF-1 in their bodies.

Diabetes

Studies in various countries have shown a strong link between the consumption of dairy products and the incidence of insulin-dependent diabetes. In 1992 researchers found that a specific dairy protein sparks an auto-immune reaction, which is believed to be what destroys the insulin-producing cells of the pancreas. Insulin is required to convert glucose from food into energy.

If the pancreas does not produce enough insulin then the glucose content in the blood is too high and diabetes occurs. Studies suggest that persons with Type 2 diabetes (non-insulin dependent diabetes) can improve and, in some cases, even reverse, the disease by switching to an unrefined vegan diet.

Dairy And Crohn's Disease

Research has linked the intestinal disorder Crohn's disease – that causes fever, diarrhea and pain after eating – with Johne's disease in dairy cows. The bacterium in cows interferes with their digestion, lowers milk production, and eventually kills those infected.

This same bacterium has been found in the gut of humans suffering from Crohn's disease, whose symptoms include crippling stomach pain, diarrhea and other intestinal problems. In addition to genetic factors and bacterial infections, Crohn's disease is affected by diet.

The Physicians Committee for Responsible Medicine (www.pcrm.org) has reported that 'many people with the illness have little fiber – specifically vegetables and fruits – and too much sugar in their diet.

Boosting plant foods, including whole grain bread and brown rice, while avoiding sugar, white flour, and white rice has reduced patient hospitalizations in research studies.'

Allergies

Consuming dairy products has also been linked to a number of allergies such as asthma, eczema and wheezing, especially in childhood. Naturally, the best beverage for infants and small toddlers is mother's breast milk. Even after the first year, food allergies to milk and milk products are common.

Many children and teens with irritable bowel syndrome, asthma, and allergies improve when they stop drinking cow's milk.

For people who suffer from Irritable Bowel Syndrome (intestinal problem), foods rich in fat such as dairy can make the symptoms worse.

Vegetarian Nutrition

Some people going vegetarian worry about getting enough protein, calcium, B vitamins and other essential nutrients. The best evidence indicates that a balanced non-animal diet is the healthiest there is – for children as well as for adults.

"Vegetarians have lower rates of obesity, coronary heart disease, high blood pressure, large bowel disorders, cancers and gall stones. Cholesterol levels tend to be lower in vegetarians." British Medical Association.

"Appropriately planned vegan and lacto-ovovegetarian diets satisfy nutrient needs of infants, children and adolescents and promote normal growth." The American Dietetic Association.

"Vegetarian groups have been shown to have lower risks of cardiovascular disease, lower rates of obesity and longer life expectancy than meat-eaters." The World Cancer Research Fund.

This section by kind permission of Animal Aid. (animalaid.org.uk).

Can Giving Up Sugar Make You Live Longer and Look Younger?

There is a growing body of evidence to suggest that consumption of sugar has a direct effect on how young or old you look for your age. Scientists from the Leiden University Medical Center in the Netherlands and manufacturing giant Unilever in the UK conducted a test involving 600 men and women aged between 50 and 70. They measured their blood sugar levels and then showed their photographs to a panel of 60 assessors who were asked to estimate how old each test subject looked.

After taking into account whether or not the test subjects smoked (which is one of the major causes of aging – give it up now!) the test showed that those with higher blood sugar levels were estimated to look older than those with lower blood sugar levels.

Sugar itself is not the aging agent, it's the way the body processes the sugar that causes the problems. Chow down a cream cake or chocolate chip cookie and your body converts that sugar to glucose, the main source of fuel for your body.

The sugar attaches itself to proteins in the body such as the collagen and elastin in the skin and produces harmful molecules called 'advanced glycation end products'. Collagen bulks out the skin to give it a younger, more plump look while elastin gives the skin 'recoil' – it's ability to return to it's original state when you frown or pinch yourself. These advanced glycation end products effect both these characteristics of skin by making skin proteins more rigid, which in turn means the skin loses it's youthful plumpness and wrinkles form more easily.

That's not the only negative effect sugar has on skin proteins. There are three different types of collagen in your skin (type one, two and three) and you need a combination of all three to keep it healthy, however sugar encourages type three collagen to morph into the more brittle type one making the skin appear thinner, more wrinkled and more susceptible to environmental and UV damage.

How much you could be effected by this glycation process depends on your diet, your age, level of fitness and metabolism. If you are a 25 year old who exercises regularly, your body will tolerate a higher level of glycation before damage occurs than a 50 year old who vegetates in front of the TV every night.

The good news is that if you start restricting your intake of sugar today, the beneficial results, such as not having such dry skin, can show quite quickly, perhaps within days.

To begin your road to recovery, avoid all the obvious sweet and tempting culprits such as cakes, cookies, candy and sweet breakfast cereals. Cut out sugary drinks and reduce your intake of high sugar alcoholic drinks such as beer. Try replacing your regular pint or bottle of beer with a glass of red wine which is not so sugar-rich.

Refined carbohydrates found in products like white bread and white rice which have a high glycaemic index because the carbohydrates within are quickly converted by the body into glucose. Replace them with brown rice, wholemeal pasta and wholemeal bread.

Also keep an eye out for hidden sugars found in cooking sauces, condiments like tomato ketchup and canned foods like baked beans. When you next go shopping, remember to read ingredients labels because sugar can be hidden in the most unlikely of food stuffs! In all, sugar should make up less than ten percent of your total diet but don't be too hard on yourself. The odd treat every now and again is unlikely to do any lasting damage.

Is Calorie Restriction the Real Fountain of Youth?

A more obvious side effect of eating too much sugar is weigh gain. But even if you don't gain weight easily, there is another negative effect of sugar to watch out for: Recent research shows a relationship between lower-calorie diets and longer life spans. For example, mice fed with half the calories they usually eat were observed to live 40 percent longer than normal while studies carried out on yeast cells, which age in much the same way as human cells, showed that their lifespan extended when glucose was restricted in their diet.

Other studies around the world have revealed that an increase in consumption of sugar also has a profound effects on your potential to develop 'old age' diseases such as Alzheimer's and cancer.

It appears that high blood glucose levels lead to a decreased level of brain activity in the hippocampus. Since the hippocampus is important for memory and learning, a decrease in brain activity here can make Alzheimer's more pronounced. It's important to note that many patients in the early stages of Alzheimer's have damage to the hippocampus region of their brain.

Research conducted at the University of Alabama in the US revealed a possible link between restricted glucose in the diet and both longer cell life and the behavior of cancers. To make this discovery, researchers fed reduced levels of glucose to laboratory-grown human lung cells and cells that were at the early stages of cancer formation.

The cells ability to grow, divide and survive was monitored over a number of weeks and researchers found that normal cells given less glucose lived longer than expected while the cells in danger of turning cancerous died before developing into full-blown cancer.

How many calories should you cut from your diet to enjoy these benefits? A study in the June 2008 issue of Rejuvenation Research, found that cutting approximately 300 to 500 calories per day from your diet had a similar biological anti-aging effect in humans as it did on mice and rats.

Here's a simple and, in the author's opinion, easy way you can restrict the amount of calories you take in on a daily basis. Make yourself a large bowl of oatmeal/porridge in the morning for breakfast. Use about 1 cup of oats and use semi skimmed or skimmed cow's milk or plant-based milks such as soy and almond. If you find porridge somewhat bland in taste, try adding mixed nuts, dried fruit or cocoa powder to the mix.

I have personally found that this keeps me feeling full and satisfied right through the day, the hunger pangs only kicking in around late afternoon. Oats provide a good source of slow release energy to keep you going throughout the day without having to snack or eat lunch.

Your body does need some sugar for energy but, as you have seen, too much may age your body in unexpected ways.

References and acknowledgements: Hegsted DM. 1986 Calcium and osteoporosis. J Nutr. 116: 2316-9.

Frank Hu et al. 1999. Dietary saturated fats and their food sources in relation to the risk of coronary heart disease in women. American Journal of Clinical Nutrition, 70: 1001-1008.

Cadogan J, Eastell R, Jones N, Barker ME. 1997. Milk intake and bone mineral acquisition in adolescent girls: randomised, controlled intervention trial. BMJ. 315:1255-69.

Karjalainen J, Martin JM, Knip M, et al. 1992. A bovine albumin peptide as a possible trigger of insulin-dependent diabetes mellitus. N Engl J Med. 327:302-7.

Nicholson AS, Sklar M, Barnard ND, et al. 1999. Toward improved management of NIDDM: A radomized, controlled, pilot intervention using a low-fat, vegetarian diet. Prev Med Aug;29 (2):87-91.

Using Your Subconscious Mind to Live Longer and Look Younger

You would think that with the billions of dollars NASA. spends on launching probes and satellites into the farthest reaches of the universe that space, as Captain James T Kirk said, was the final frontier. I beg to differ. I suggest to you it is 'inner space', the human mind, than represents a greater enigma than the distant stars ever will.

Thanks to modern technology, our knowledge of the external has, much like the universe itself, expanded rapidly. We can be certain of the motions of the planets around far off suns and have discovered that an insubstantial 'dark matter' fills the heavens, yet the grey matter between our ears still remains somewhat of a mystery.

So what do we know? We know your mind is incredible and has been described as a biological computer more powerful than any electronic brain yet devised by man. Every man made thing we see around us, from the smallest ball bearing to gigantic Apollo space rockets, was first conceived in and then made reality by the human mind.

Although all our man-made achievements may seem impressive, it is generally accepted that we use only about 10% of the brain's ability, whilst the remaining 90% remains dormant and unused.

That part we have used to create our world demonstrates only a fraction of the human mind's capabilities. What we have discovered and achieved so far is only the tip of the proverbial iceberg.

To Boldly Go

Of this we are certain. If you were to compare the mind to Captain Kirk's Starship Enterprise you'd see there were two things going on at the same time as it speeds through space.

First you have the crew, busying themselves with the everyday tasks needed to keep everything ship shape. This is like the conscious mind, the part you are using now to read these words and over which we have most control. We use it for daily decision making, rational thinking and other everyday tasks.

But your average starship crewman probably doesn't think about all the other unseen, unnoticed things going on in the ship that keep him alive and prevent the ship from slamming into asteroids.

There's the air conditioning that lets him breathe and keeps the temperature just right. There's the lifts speeding people to other decks, doors opening and shutting automatically to let him in and out of rooms, and millions of routine computer processes that every second keep the ship and its crew 'alive' and functioning normally.

Similarly the subconscious takes care of all the automatic functions we need to stay alive but which we don't have to think about every second of the day, such as breathing (you don't have to think "now I breathe in, now I breathe out" do you?), emotions, imagination, memories and the autonomic nervous system - pupil dilation, saliva production, skin condition, that sort of thing. Two different ships, two different 'yous' inhabiting the same space, interdependent on each other and subtly interacting all day and all night.

And, like the computers on the Enterprise, the subconscious also possesses the remarkable ability to record everything you've seen, heard, experienced or learned since you were born, even things you were not consciously aware of at the time. You may not be able to access that information right now but it's all in there somewhere. That's why police forces around the world sometimes use professional hypnotherapists to hypnotise crime scene witnesses.

Under hypnosis the conscious mind is 'bypassed' and the subconscious 'tape recorder' accessed to recall photographic details about a scene that, at the time, the witness may not have consciously registered.

Tell the computer on Enterprise to blow up the ship and it will probably do it, no questions asked. It doesn't reason or question the command. Same with the subconscious - it records anything and everything and believes whatever it is told, if it is told often enough.

That's bad if you keep telling it you are useless or unworthy or fat or not loveable or whatever that little niggling negative voice inside all of us keeps saying. The subconscious just says "okay, that's fine, so be it" and will do its utmost to make those beliefs come true. But what if you were to keep telling it "you are great, you are self confident, you are loveable and you are slim"? Same thing, subconscious accepts these things to be true and will change your belief systems, way of acting and re-acting to the outside world accordingly.

The subconscious cannot resist consistent bombardment of one simple idea or set of instructions. It simply has to give in and give you whatever you want. The subconscious is that powerful! Not convinced? Take these examples.

Perhaps one of the most often quoted and well known examples of the incredible power of the subconscious mind was an experiment carried out in the 1950's on a cinema audience in America.

During the movie, just a single frame with the simple instruction to buy a certain product, was inserted into the film. As a single frame it flashed by without the viewers even noticing it was there but sure enough, come the interval, everyone went out to the bar and bought the product and overall sales soared!

Luckily, so effective was this form of subconscious advertising, it was banned before any other company could jump on the bandwagon and bend unsuspecting audiences to its commercial will. Still, the fantastic power of this method to influence the way people think and act did not escape the British and American medical authorities who, in the same decade, gave official approval for the use of hypnosis in treating both physical and psychological disorders.

Since then, the amazing ability of the mind to control both physical and mental states has been proven again and again. Doctors and therapists all over the world recognise hypnosis as a valuable therapeutic tool that can be used to treat asthma, tension, headaches, stomach disorders, blood pressure, smoking and many other physical ailments.

Even dentists are now using a form of hypnosis on patients so that they feel no pain during treatment without having to take a conventional anaesthetic.

Boosting the health of the body is one of the areas where hypnosis seems to work particularly well. Years of clinical research and controlled experiments seem to suggest that it is possible to boost your immune system just by thinking about it.

Nicholas Hall, a neurophysiologist at George Washington University Medical Center in America found that his subjects could increase the number of white blood cells, as well as an immunity hormone called Thymosin-alpha-1, in their bloodstream by simply using visualization exercises.

Still not convinced? Try this one for size. At the University of Texas, Dr Frank Lawlis found that if his subjects used their imaginations in a creative way, they could boost the number of disease fighting cells, called Neutrofils, in their bloodstream.

Similarly, in Japan, doctors found in controlled tests that their subjects could eliminate the itching, swelling and blistering caused by exposure to a poisonous plant by imagining, under hypnosis, that it was harmless. Amazingly, when the experiment was reversed and patients were told that a harmless plant was poisonous, their skin reacted as if they had really been exposed to its harmful chemicals!

This, to me, demonstrates beyond doubt the power of the mind to influence the body. If it can have this much influence on our physical state, just imagine what it can do for our mental one! The subconscious mind also has enormous influence over what way we think. It affects the way we feel, the way we see the world and the way we deal with life.

What is Hypnosis?

When I talk about hypnosis I don't mean the silly kind you see on television where some stage hypnotist makes a poor unsuspecting victim believe he's Mr Spock and has no control over his actions (although this is another good example of how the subconscious can be made to modify your belief and behavior). I'm talking about hypnotherapy, which is another kettle of fish altogether but often confused with the kind used for entertainment.

Hypnosis in this context does not mean someone completely taking control of your mind and turning you into some kind of zombie to provide embarrassing entertainment for audiences. It could be compared more accurately to a pleasant bout of daydreaming. It's not like going to sleep and you do not become unconscious. You are still aware of your surroundings to some extent and are still in charge of all your faculties so no-one can make you bark like a dog if you don't want to!

Instead you feel pleasantly relaxed but mentally alert. Hypnosis is a very pleasant, relaxing state to be in because your consciousness is directed inwards so you become comfortably detached from the outside world.

You could say it's a 'shift' in consciousness, where the inner imaginary world comes more to the fore and the everyday reality of life is relegated to the back of your mind.

It is in this state that the subconscious mind becomes much more susceptible to either negative or positive suggestion. It makes no distinction between the two.

Why? Because hypnosis bypasses our conscious, reasoning, skeptical, disbelieving mind set and speaks directly to the non-judgemental, easily fooled, all trusting subconscious. Here's what the Encyclopaedia Britannica has to say on the subject.

"Hypnosis is defined as a special psychological state with certain physiological attributes resembling sleep only superficially and marked by a functioning of the individual at a level of awareness other than the ordinary conscious state.
This state is characterised by a degree of increased receptiveness and responsiveness in which inner perceptions are given as much significance as is generally given only to external reality".

> For more anti-aging tips go to
> goodallcopywriting.com and
> visit the blog.

A Little bit of History

The word 'hypnosis' was coined in the 19th century but it is a very ancient form of behavioral therapy. The ancient Sumerian civilization which existed about 4000 years BCE were using hypnosis as a therapeutic tool as did Hindu Fakirs, Persian Magi, Indian Yogis, the physicians of ancient Egypt and healers of the middle ages.

Perhaps one of the most famous practitioners of the art was a German physician called Franz Anton Mesmer who lived from 1784 to 1815. Although his strange techniques were in pseudo mystery and amateur dramatics, he never realized that when he transfixed his patients into a kind of trance, he was using a form of hypnosis. His legacy lives on to this day in the word 'Mesmerized' which is still used to describe a form of hypnotic influence.

But it wasn't until the 18th century that an English optometrist called James Braid observed that a trance-like state could be achieved when a person fixed their gaze on a shining object for a few minutes and coined the term 'hypnosis', which comes from the Greek word 'hypnos' for sleep. As we have seen, during hypnosis you don't really fall asleep so the name is somewhat inaccurate but, for better or worse, it has stuck.

Today, all over the world, professional hypnotherapists are helping people overcome physical problems or modify their thinking and behavior, and transforming lives for the better using this truly ancient form of therapy.

The great news is that you don't have to go and visit a therapist (and pay their high fees) to benefit from this remarkable self-help system, you can transform your life from the comfort of your own armchair or bed.

If life is too busy even to squeeze in 30 minutes of uninterrupted relaxation, listening to subliminal suggestions while driving to work, at the gym, or doing the household chores works equally as well.

These subliminal suggestions are commonly masked under some pleasant music or natural sounds such as crashing waves. The great thing about this is that you can go about your daily business just listening to the music in the background but all the time your subconscious is absorbing those positive suggestions.

It is also a great way for sceptics to enjoy the benefits of self-hypnosis, even if they don't believe it works. Self-hypnosis works in spite of your beliefs to the contrary.

You don't have to try and 'make' it work. Your subconscious believes whatever you tell it. It's the perfect 'no effort' way to change you for the better.

If, on the other hand, you like the idea of having a quiet and relaxing 30 minutes to yourself, use the auditory version of those same suggestions either when your are drifting off to sleep or when you feel like a relaxing break.

In the beginning, you might be asked to use your imagination to conjure up a relaxing visualization exercise that will help you drift off into a pleasant daydream-like state while the positive suggestions are repeated over and over to you on a conscious level.

There's nothing magical or occult about this, just one of the most relaxing, pleasant and comfortable experiences you can have that gives you control over your mind and body not normally available in your normal, conscious state.

In this relaxed frame of mind the suggestions are more readily accepted because the critical faculties of the conscious mind are partially suspended, allowing the suggestions to be delivered to the non-judgemental subconscious mind for storage.

There are potentially huge benefits for you if you use hypnosis as part of your everyday life. When you understand hypnosis you start to see its potential to improve human performance physically, emotionally and intellectually.

So you see, it's not outer space that poses some of the greatest challenges we have ever faced, it's inner space. Your mind is the 'final frontier' just waiting to be explored and exploited for your ultimate benefit.

How Can Hypnosis Help Me Look and Feel Younger?

There definitely are things you can do with hypnosis that will help you reduce the effects of aging. For example, when you relax very deeply, you can alter the blood flow to different areas of the body, relax muscles at will, decrease your blood pressure, boost your immune system and change deep-seated attitudes. And all this without a needle in sight!

Old fashioned self hypnosis cassette tapes have been around for many years. I've been using them since the 1970's to great effect but recent technological breakthroughs have taken this wonderful method of self-transformation to a whole new level with CD's and MP3 downloads.

These anti-aging hypnosis downloads will help give you the best chance of staying fit and trim and healthy and young at heart.

How to Cope Confidently With Hair Loss/Thinning

Hair loss or thinning of the hair is a common consequence of aging and there are plenty of products and businesses out there offering you life-like wigs, hair transplants or chemicals you massage into your scalp that are supposed to stimulate hair growth.

Whilst hypnosis may not be able to make your hair grow back overnight, it can help you with worries about your receding hair line, make you feel less self-conscious about your hair, and revive your self-confidence about the way you look.

Accepting hair loss is an audio hypnosis session prepared by experienced psychologists that will help you really relax around the idea that you are losing your hair.

Learn more about this hypnosis course at:

Set Your Unconscious Mind to Live Longer

Although diet, exercise and genetics play a big role in how long you live and how healthy you are, many studies have shown that your attitude toward aging is also a key factor in longevity.

We've all heard of stories where an authority figure such as a doctor has given a patient six months to live. The patient goes away and their belief in this prognosis is so strong, they expire exactly six months later, not because the outcome was certain (the doctor may only have been estimating the time they had left), but because the patient's belief in the outcome was so strong.
The mind made it come true for them. But suggestion of this kind can work in the opposite direction too.

Research conducted at Hull University in the UK demonstrated that cancer patients who received hypnotherapy appeared to live significantly longer than those who didn't have the hypnosis.

The 'placebo effect' is well known in the healing arts. A placebo is something that has no effect on the body, such as a sugar pill, but the patient is told it is a new wonder drug that can cure their illness.

Because the patient believes what he or she has been told, the placebo sometimes has the same or even greater effect than the drug.

Dr John Hagelin, a quantum physicist and public policy expert has also recognised the link between mind and body:

"Our body is really the product of our thoughts. We're beginning to understand in medical science the degree to which the nature of thoughts and emotions actually determines the physical substance and structure and function of our bodies."

And there are many other pieces of research showing the impact of optimism on health. The 'Set your mind to live longer' MP3 will help you develop a positive, energetic attitude to life as you age, making sure that your mind has the right blueprint for an active healthy later life.

Learn more about this hypnosis course at:

http://www.hypnosisdownloads.com/anti-aging/live-longer?4405

For more anti-aging tips go to
goodallcopywriting.com and
visit the blog.

Get a Natural Anti-Aging Attitude

The thought of getting older can be depressing, especially if you associate it with negative images such as slowing down, getting weaker, feeling more frail and over the hill. Trouble is, the more we think these things and focus on them, the more they will come into our life because the subconscious mind will simply deliver to you that which you always think about.

But it doesn't have to be this way. Research shows that having positive ideas about aging can affect the rate at which you age and how you age.

There are many examples of men in their 70's, 80's and older who are still as active, fit and sharp as guys half their age and who still has a great sense of humour and zest for life.

Our society is obsessed with youth but 'youth' is a concept that can be separated from how many years you happen to have clocked up! 'Youth' is an attitude, a state of mind and you can continue to develop socially, physically and in all ways as you grow older.

Learn more about this hypnosis course at:

http://www.hypnosisdownloads.com/anti-aging/anti-aging?4405

Get a Non-Surgical Face Lift Using Hypnosis

Considering a face-lift? Before you go under the knife or reach for the syringe, consider what both The Five Minute Face Lift Workout and a non-surgical face lift using hypnosis could do for you. Did you know that stress and tension is one of the major causes of lines and wrinkles?

Stress, tension and worry cause frequent frowning which, over time, cause the muscles in the face to conform to that movement thanks to 'muscle memory'. That's why they call those forehead wrinkles 'worry lines'.

Hypnotherapists have noticed for years that after a session of deep hypnosis people invariably look fresher and younger with smoother skin. In the *'Non-Surgical Face Lift'* hypnosis download session you'll experience a kind of natural lift and rejuvenation as your sub-conscious mind is encouraged to relax all the muscles of your face and circulation is encouraged into the skin of the face. You will also be given powerful suggestions to do more of what helps your skin such as drinking more water and eating good foods.

Learn more about this hypnosis course at:

http://www.hypnosisdownloads.com/anti-aging/face-lift?4405

Conclusion

If you want to 'stop the clock' on the signs of aging and stop wrinkles, this book will show you a quick, natural and easy way to not being a victim of time, and instead become it's master.

Like you, I began to notice the effects of the passage of time whenever I looked in the mirror - the frown lines, the crow's feet, the eye bags, the dropping mouth and the sagging skin. Quite frankly it depressed me.

Like everyone else, I thought that the gradual decline in my appearance was just something I would have to learn to live with and resigned myself to the accompanying loss of self-esteem and self-confidence.

That was until I discovered this surprisingly simple and natural way to stop and even reverse facial aging and look years younger.

I'm excited to reveal this amazing exercise system that can rapidly roll back the years and breathe new life into your face:

Is the chance of rolling back the years and regaining some of your lost youth worth investing just a few minutes of your time?

Enjoy the journey and let me know how you get on.

Simon.